THIRD EDITION

UNDERSTANDING THE WORK OF
Nurse Theorists
A Creative Beginning

Kathleen Sitzman, PhD, RN, CNE, ANEF
Professor
Undergraduate–Senior
East Carolina University
Greenville, North Carolina

Lisa Wright Eichelberger, PhD, RN
Dean and Professor, College of Health
Clayton State University
Atlanta, Georgia

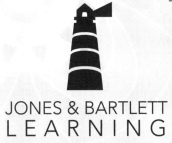

JONES & BARTLETT
LEARNING

World Headquarters
Jones & Bartlett Learning
5 Wall Street
Burlington, MA 01803
978-443-5000
info@jblearning.com
www.jblearning.com

Jones & Bartlett Learning books and products are available through most bookstores and online booksellers. To contact Jones & Bartlett Learning directly, call 800-832-0034, fax 978-443-8000, or visit our website, www.jblearning.com.

Substantial discounts on bulk quantities of Jones & Bartlett Learning publications are available to corporations, professional associations, and other qualified organizations. For details and specific discount information, contact the special sales department at Jones & Bartlett Learning via the above contact information or send an email to specialsales@jblearning.com.

09807-5

Production Credits
Chief Executive Officer: Ty Field
President: James Homer
Chief Product Officer: Eduardo Moura
VP, Executive Publisher: David D. Cella
Executive Editor: Amanda Martin
Acquisitions Editor: Teresa Reilly
Editorial Assistant: Lauren Vaughn
Production Manager: Carolyn Rogers Pershouse
Production Assistant: Juna Abrams
VP of Marketing: Alisha Weisman
Senior Marketing Manager: Jennifer Scherzay
VP, Manufacturing and Inventory Control:
   Therese Connell
Composition: CAE Solutions Corp.
Cover Design: Michael O'Donnell
Rights & Media Research Assistant: Wes DeShano
Media Development Editor: Shannon Sheehan
Cover and Title Page Image: © Irmairma/Shutterstock
Printing and Binding: Edwards Brothers Malloy
Cover Printing: Edwards Brothers Malloy

Library of Congress Cataloging-in-Publication Data
Sitzman, Kathleen, author.
  Understanding the work of nurse theorists : a creative beginning / Kathleen L. Sitzman, Lisa Wright Eichelberger. -- Third edition.
    p. ; cm.
  Includes bibliographical references and index.
  ISBN 978-1-284-09150-2 (paperback)
  I. Eichelberger, Lisa Wright, author. II. Title.
  [DNLM: 1. Nursing Theory. 2. Models, Nursing. WY 86]
  RT84.5
  610.73--dc23
                            2015021057

6048

Printed in the United States of America
19 18 17 16 15   10 9 8 7 6 5 4 3 2 1

Dedication

I would like to dedicate this work to my husband, Rick, and to the rest of my family. Thank you for your love and unwavering support.

—Kathleen L. Sitzman

First of all, I would like to express my deep gratitude to Dr. Kathy Sitzman, my writing partner and friend. Her sweet spirit is a rare and mighty thing, and our third edition of this textbook would not have happened without her understanding and support. Thank you, Kathy.

To my husband John, your love, care, and devotion during our lifetime together has given me true joy. Elaine says thanks!

Karen, there is no one closer to me than you. Thanks for sharing my past, present, and future. Let's hear it for the "Wright Girls."

To my children, what can I say? I am so proud of each of you. You make my heart sing! Thank you especially for giving us the next generation of little Eichelbergers, Riley, Neila, Everett, and John Mason. I can't wait to watch them soar!

And, finally, to Dr. Jean Kelley and the faculty at the University of Alabama School of Nursing, University of Alabama at Birmingham. You opened my eyes to the wonderful world of nursing theory. You gave me the chance to study with actual nurse theorists and be challenged by them. Even today, in my mind, this young student is still inspired by their words.

—Lisa Wright Eichelberger

Contents

FOREWORD ix

PREFACE xi

Part I
Introduction to Theory in Nursing

1 WHAT IS NURSING THEORY? 3

2 WHY ARE THEORIES IMPORTANT IN NURSING? 7

3 THE DEVELOPMENT OF NURSING THEORIES 11

4 EVALUATING A THEORY 19

Part II
Theories That Define Nursing or Discuss Nursing in a General Sense: Philosophies

5 USING THE ART OF GEORGES SEURAT TO ENVISION PHILOSOPHIES 25

6 FLORENCE NIGHTINGALE'S DEFINITION OF NURSING 29

7 VIRGINIA HENDERSON'S DEFINITION OF NURSING 35

8 ERNESTINE WIEDENBACH'S HELPING ART OF CLINICAL NURSING 41

9 JEAN WATSON'S THEORY OF HUMAN/TRANSPERSONAL CARING 47

Part III
Theories About Broad Nursing Practice Areas: Grand Theories

10	ENVISIONING THEORIES THROUGH MANDALA ART	65
11	MYRA ESTRIN LEVINE'S CONSERVATION MODEL	69
12	BETTY NEUMAN'S SYSTEMS MODEL	75
13	SISTER CALLISTA ROY'S ADAPTATION MODEL	81
14	DOROTHEA OREM'S SELF-CARE MODEL	89
15	MADELEINE LEININGER'S CULTURE CARE: DIVERSITY AND UNIVERSALITY THEORY	95

Part IV
Theories About Specific Nursing Actions, Processes, or Concepts: Middle-Range Theories

16	ENVISIONING THEORIES THROUGH ORIGAMI ART	105
17	IDA JEAN ORLANDO-PELLETIER'S NURSING PROCESS THEORY	111
18	KATHARINE KOLCABA'S THEORY OF COMFORT	117
19	NOLA PENDER'S HEALTH-PROMOTION MODEL	125
20	HILDEGARD PEPLAU'S INTERPERSONAL RELATIONS IN NURSING	137
21	IMOGENE KING'S CONCEPTUAL SYSTEM AND THEORY OF GOAL ATTAINMENT	143
22	PATRICIA BENNER'S MODEL OF SKILL ACQUISITION IN NURSING	155
23	AFAF IBRAHIM MELEIS'S TRANSITIONS THEORY	165

Part V
Theories That Defy Classification

24 Envisioning Theories That Defy Classification Through Space Photography 179

25 Martha Rogers's Unitary Human Beings 181

26 Margaret Newman's Health as Expanding Consciousness 187

27 Rosemarie Rizzo Parse's Theory of Human Becoming 193

Part VI
Conclusion

28 Further Development of Nursing Theory 205

29 Use of Information Technology by Nurse Theorists 209

30 Twentieth Anniversary of Nursing Theory on the World Wide Web 217

Glossary 227

Index 229

Foreword

This work in nursing theory opens new doors and opens up new horizons of learning, studying, embodying, and using nursing theory. It is an introduction to creative scholarship, inviting new, engaging, artistic, aesthetic, imaginary, and evocative approaches to entering into, and participating in, inspirited and inspired learning. Understanding the Work of Nurse Theorists: A Creative Beginning takes us into new territory for teaching and learning theory, while interacting with the depth of philosophical, idealistic, ethical, theoretical constructs, concepts, and meanings embedded in diverse theories. This unique and original approach to nursing theory is not otherwise offered when considering learning and teaching nursing theory.

Sitzman and Eichelberger have a special grasp and postmodern view of the significance and insights that can be gained from diverse approaches to learning that draw upon all ways of knowing, being, and learning. They offer an original pedagogical perspective that integrates art and artistry with concepts and methods of thinking while probing philosophical insights through concrete, original, creative-artistic learning experiences and exercises that bring theory to life and make it a living process. By doing so, readers and students cocreate the learning–discovery process.

This text opens the hearts and minds of readers and students to let in fresh air and present new ways of learning. The text of theory is to be read as an open, evolving text rather than a closed, set, stable subject.

This text takes us into the heart of the theorists' thinking, while assisting the student with self-created challenges to use creativity, curiosity, thoughtfulness, and joy of discovery. The authors help to illuminate new depths of learning for seeing the relevance and dynamic living nature of theory-in-action in our personal/professional lives and work. It is a book that takes us into the new world of learning and teaching, beyond the sterile rote, staid thinking that often dominates our views of theory.

It is through works such as this that nurses will learn that they are the theories; theories are not separate and detached from their being but are a living thought system that both informs and guides nursing into this new century, while sustaining the finest of the historical heritage and roots of nursing. *Understanding the Work of Nurse Theorists: A Creative Beginning* is a book for beginners and experts alike, inspiriting and inspiring a new generation of students, nurses, theorists, and theories.

Jean Watson, PhD, RN, HNC, FAAN
Distinguished Professor of Nursing
Murchinson-Scoville Chair of Caring Science
University of Colorado Health Sciences Center

Preface

Nursing theories are the creative products of nurses who seek to thoughtfully describe relationships and interactions that exist within nursing practice. Theories address the many questions that confront nurses daily. Theories are multilayered and consist of numerous tangible and intangible components. Attempts at initial understanding of complex nursing theories are often overwhelming and intensely unsatisfying for beginning students.

Most undergraduate nursing students are exposed to nursing theory in a limited way during the process of completing basic nursing education. Unfortunately, the attitude of students taking nursing theory for the first time is often one of dread. Many express the opinion that theory has little relevance for present or future clinical practice. Often, it becomes the task of nursing educators to try and convey the idea that theory is important for the continued growth and development of nursing practice. This text is designed for first-time nursing theory students who may believe that theory will be irrelevant, uninspiring, and difficult to grasp.

When beginning the study of nursing theory, two things must be made clear to students:

1. Nursing theory is relevant to present and future practice.
2. Students are not expected to become nurse theorists or experts.

Traditional theory teaching methods have not always been effective in communicating the above two points to students. In theory classes, papers and other writing-based projects often are assigned in which the student is required to somehow comprehend the complex web of ideas that constitutes nursing theory and then expound on how theory informs practice or applies to personal professional experience. Producing coherent assignments about nursing theory requires a relatively advanced level of understanding that may not be accessible to students with limited exposure to the material. Students expend a great deal of energy in the struggle to produce "perfect" assignments with acceptable levels of understanding, and in the course of this struggle, teaching/learning opportunities to draw the student in, to experience the gestalt and beauty of nursing theory, melt away. After struggling through what often seems to be an exercise in confusion and futility, many students vow never to study nursing theory again after formal education is complete.

Most currently available theory texts are more complex and detailed than what is needed, or desired, for classes taught at the beginning level, and therefore, may be more confusing than helpful for most students. Unfortunately, this often leads to either frustrated students and instructors or (in response to the frustration) the elimination of all but cursory content at the baccalaureate level. If students are instead encouraged to approach the challenge of comprehending nursing theory from the position of a beginner's mind, with creativity, curiosity, thoughtfulness, and joy, then the learning process has the power to clarify and illuminate depths of nursing theory in ways that will hold meaning for the student long after the class is over.

This text offers a different approach to teaching and learning nursing theory. The essential definitions and basic concepts are presented along with a brief overview of the most common nursing theories. However, what is unique about this text is the use of art to illuminate nursing theories. This method mobilizes creativity for the construction of personal meaning. In encouraging creativity through the use of the universal language of art, students become engaged and active learners. When this text and learning activities are used as a guide for learning, students do not sit passively in a classroom, memorizing definitions and facts. The activities outlined in this text are visual, tactile, and kinesthetic. Students are able to read, see, touch, and manipulate the learning materials. Although comprehensive understanding of theory (perfect understanding) is not the intent or result of this creative approach, a light of beginning understanding will be ignited by this approach.

A quote by Leonard Cohen says it well:

> Ring the bells that still can ring,
> forget your perfect offering.
> There is a crack in everything.
> That's how the light gets in.*

Another way to explain this creative approach is the chocolate chip cookie example. As with nursing theory, a chocolate chip cookie consists of numerous components, both tangible (i.e., color, texture, size) and intangible (i.e., how tempting it may look to the casual passerby).

***Anthem**
Words and Music by Leonard Cohen
Copyright (c) 1992 Sony/ATV Music Publishing LLC and Stranger Music Inc.
All Rights Administered by Sony/ATV Music Publishing LLC, 424 Church Street, Suite 1200, Nashville, TN 37219
International Copyright Secured   All Rights Reserved
Reprinted by Permission of Hal Leonard Corporation

To convey a complete understanding of all that is a chocolate chip cookie, a teacher might thoroughly describe, diagram, and explain down to the chemical and atomic levels exactly what one is. The information obtained during this type of teaching/learning exchange would be undoubtedly accurate in every detail. Unfortunately, if the student has never tasted a chocolate chip cookie, the prospect of trying to appreciate and understand one seems, at best, bewildering and, at worst, frustrating busywork. And so it is with the introductory study of nursing theory.

The alternative learning methods suggested in this handbook offer beginning opportunities for learning through visual and experiential pathways, similar to tasting a cookie before studying it in depth. The methods are also meant to support personal discovery and the construction of individual meaning, for instance, "This cookie tastes pretty interesting! I want to learn more!" This is a somewhat back-door approach to generating learning moments by offering glimpses of the complete picture before attempting to dissect and understand the complexity of the components. Most nursing theories are unquestionably complex; however, simplicity of explanation is used in this text to foster freedom of thought and creativity and to draw the student in so that in-depth study will be more willingly embraced later.

Introduction to Theory in Nursing

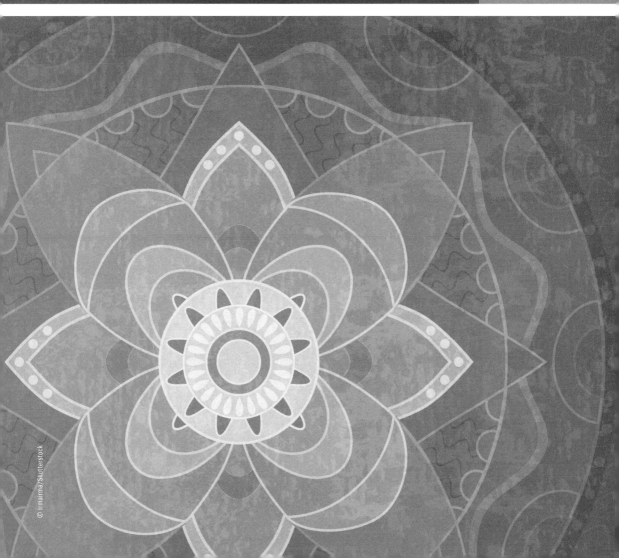

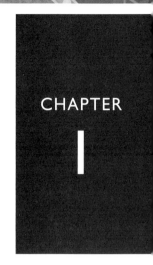

CHAPTER

1

What Is Nursing Theory?

Nursing theories are the creative products of nurses who seek (or sought) to thoughtfully describe the many aspects of nursing in ways that could be studied, evaluated, and used by other nurses. In other words, theory is an attempt to explain patterns and relationships found in nursing phenomena. Nurse theorists are people who are or have been nurses, have thought deeply about how one might describe the phenomenon of nursing, and then have tried in their own way, from their own perspective, to record their thoughts and observations based on professional and personal experiences. Each theory is as unique as the individual(s) who created it.

In many cases, the creators of nursing theories did not set out to "become" nurse theorists. For the most part, theories evolved, and continue to evolve, out of creative attempts to describe nursing phenomena in ways that made sense to the theorists and others. Published nursing theories stimulate formal debate, exploration, and research regarding the nature and process of nursing. Theories give nurses different ways of viewing reality, such as expanding awareness of concepts never before considered, organizing care activities, and providing opportunities for reflection and the formation of opinions. Nursing theories are formal tools for communication that enable experienced nurses to communicate specific perceptions about nursing in a structured way so that others have an opportunity to study, evaluate, participate in, and add to an ongoing dialogue meant to address questions such as:

- What do nurses do?
- What makes nursing unique from other healthcare-related professions?
- What is wholistic nursing care?
- What is meant by terms such as *wellness* and *illness*?
- Do certain nursing actions measurably improve client outcomes?
- What differentiates excellent nursing care from marginal nursing care?
- Is nursing a job, a vocation, a profession, or a combination of all three?
- Is the core of nursing "caring" or technical skill mastery?
- Is nursing meant to be an independent profession or an auxiliary component of the medical profession?
- Should nursing practice formally encompass the metaphysical? Spiritual?
- How should phenomena that cannot be concretely measured through the five senses be addressed in nursing?

These are only a few of a myriad of questions and concerns addressed by nursing theories. The focus of a particular theory depends on the concurrent historical/political/social/professional environment and the personal and professional experiences of the theorist. Because there are wide-ranging issues associated with nursing practice, theories may be created to address broad or very narrow aspects of the profession.

For the purposes of organization and ease of understanding, nursing theories can be placed into three loosely defined categories:

1. Definitions of nursing in general (philosophies)
2. Discussions of broad nursing practice areas (grand theories)
3. Assertions about specific nursing actions, processes, or concepts (middle-range theories)

Some nursing theories may fit into more than one category, depending on how they are interpreted and used by individuals. There is no firm rule regarding what category a specific theory fits into. In fact, there is much debate surrounding theory development and evaluation. The questions and ambiguity surrounding these ongoing debates may be disconcerting to those new to the study of theory because there never seems to be a *correct* answer or viewpoint. The first assignment in any study of nursing theory should be to become comfortable with ambiguity. For example, there are ongoing debates over categorical determinations or differences in terms, such as *theory* versus *model* versus *theoretical framework*. There will probably never be a final resolution to these debates because the great variety of viewpoints among nursing scholars only continues professional dialogues that stimulate exploration and learning. Because ambiguity is quite often a feature of the study of nursing theory, productive learning approaches include listening, evaluating, reading, adopting another's position to assess personal fit, formulating an informed opinion, and realizing that firm answers do not always apply.

Informed opinion based on scholarly study *is* a valid approach in deciding what category a theory might fit into at any given time. A scholar, whether beginning or expert, is expected to have an opinion based on logical, rational thought that can be explained. Making informed judgments about theories may seem a daunting task for a beginner. Methods for making such determinations will be discussed in Chapter 4. More complete discussions and examples of theory categories are contained in Parts II, III, and IV. Be aware that this text is just one approach for "making sense" of nursing theories. Use the broad categories and definitions presented here or other classification systems with the awareness that there will be variations and debates within the literature regarding nursing theory. Continued debates, however, do not diminish the importance of nursing theory for the profession. As a matter of fact, nursing theory, and its role in nursing research, has done more to advance the scholarship of nursing over the last 40 years than any other nursing endeavor. Nursing theory has served as a framework for inquiry that has allowed the profession to create its own body of knowledge. For now, it may be helpful to remember that theories, though to some extent abstract and ambiguous, exist to help nurses explain and guide the very real practice world around them.

Why Are Theories Important in Nursing?

Theories provide structure and order for guiding and improving professional practice, teaching and learning activities, and research. Exactly how might a theory be important for everyday nursing activities? Surely theories are too far removed from "nurses in the trenches" to really impact much of anything, right? This may not be necessarily so, as demonstrated by the examples in this chapter.

The following is an example of a theory influencing professional practice.

Assume a practicing nurse learns about a nursing theory that describes the "whole" of nursing practice as consisting of activities in technical, ethical, and wholistic care areas. Before learning about this theory, the nurse had focused the bulk of his/her professional effort on mastering technical skills. After learning about this theory, the nurse actively explores ethical and wholistic care concerns by reading articles about these topics in two professional journals that are delivered monthly to his/her home and by searching for related information on the Internet. The inclusion of ethical and wholistic principles into professional practice enriches personal job satisfaction and effectiveness. Client satisfaction also improves. The nurse shares information about this theory and how it has the potential to enrich professional practice with a few colleagues. Pretty soon, the nursing staff on the medical unit where the nurse works decides to adopt the theory as a formal guide for unit-wide practice. It will also be shared during orientation of new nursing staff and will be used as a guide when decisions are made regarding unit practices and policies.

The following is an example of how theories might influence teaching and learning activities.

A small university is constructing a nursing program that will provide an RN to BSN degree in nursing to qualified students who complete the program of study. There are numerous ways of teaching nursing, and there are thousands of textbooks, computer programs, and study formats to consider when constructing a program. What classes will be offered and in what order? What is the most important, central concept that all students should come away with when the course of study is completed? To clarify what direction to take in developing this program, educators will need to first decide what theories will guide educational practices. Most nursing programs in the United States base programs on one or more nursing theories, in addition to basic educational theories. In the case of this small university, it is decided to base the curriculum on three theories: two broad nursing theories that identify "wholistic caring" as the central concept in nursing practice and one other, more specific theory that describes a sequential process by which nurses may effectively provide "hands-on" client care. After selecting these theories as a guide, it then becomes possible to consciously create a course of study focused on the principles of "caring" put forth in the first two selected theories, with the third, more specific theory providing a framework for selecting and sequencing course material.

The following is an example of how a theory might guide a research activity.

Theories often provide the basis for the creation of questions that will be asked during research activities. Theories may also clarify ways in which to *focus* observations and data collection. For example, Jordan, a nurse in the newborn intensive care unit (NICU), wishes to learn if mothers who are allowed unlimited visiting time with their infants experience more effective mother–infant bonding than do mothers who are asked to adhere to a restricted visiting schedule. Jordan discovers that there are several nursing journal articles about mother–infant bonding research studies, and as a result of these past studies, theories have been created to describe the process of successful mother–infant bonding. Jordan finds one theory that makes the most sense in terms of personal professional experience and uses it as a guide in creating her study. The theory Jordan selects describes an eight-step process of bonding that starts with the mother's realization of pregnancy and culminates in successful postpartum bonding between mother and infant. Jordan decides to observe for the presence of these eight steps when assessing the progress of bonding in both groups of mothers and infants (unrestricted vs. restricted visiting). During the course of the study, Jordan may find that the eight steps described in the previous study accurately describe what is observed (validating the theory) or the eight steps may not apply at all to what is observed (not supporting the theory). In either instance, Jordan will be performing two vital functions associated with nursing research: gathering data that may be helpful in clarifying mother–infant bonding for NICU clients and assessing the validity and applicability of a previously created nursing theory. If Jordan's study validates the eight-step process, this might provide support for use of this theory for the development of programs that will support optimal mother–infant bonding in multiple NICU settings. If Jordan's study does not support the eight-step process, then valuable information regarding directions for future studies will be provided.

In a general sense, theory development supports independence of the nursing profession by creating forums where nurses have opportunities to develop and support unique professional visions. Theories specific to nursing help differentiate nursing from other care-related professions. Because nursing encompasses a variety of professional activities, there is room for a corresponding variety of nursing theories, all meant to accurately describe nursing in one way or another.

A logical question at this point might be, "Is it possible to firmly determine which theories are *correct*?" Because scholarly, well-educated nurses have created these theories, does it mean that others must accept them as truth? Just because there is a significant body of research and publications using a particular nursing theory in practice does not mean that this theory is right for every nurse.

Likewise, there is no single theory, or group of theories, that is more correct than another. Nursing practice is inexorably tied to human interactions and experiences; precise and unwavering conclusions are often not possible.

It is up to the individual to determine if a particular theory makes sense after evaluation and comparison with personal values and belief systems and if it adds value to education, practice, and research. In other words, it is the responsibility of each nurse to independently evaluate if a given theory resonates with personal professional practice. What feels "correct" for one nurse may not necessarily feel "correct" for another nurse.

Also, nurses and nursing theories are dynamic, shifting, growing entities; therefore, a theory that did not initially seem important to an individual nurse may become more important as the nurse matures or as the theory evolves through time. Usefulness of a particular theory is strongly related to personal and professional relevance at any given point in time.

Please be aware that it takes courage and vision to present to the world beliefs (theories) based on professional observations. Even if you do not agree with or appreciate a particular theory, please respect the intellect, introspection, and tremendous amount of work it took for the theorist to create a formal presentation of ideas for you to evaluate. Each model or theory is a representation of creativity and diversity within nursing ranks. In diversity there can be strength if we allow ourselves to celebrate the unique (and equally valid) visions of our colleagues that make up the totality of nursing.

The Development of Nursing Theories

The Nurse Theorists

M ost nurse theorists did not set out to create a nursing theory. Most began constructing a theory as a way to improve the care delivered to clients, whether through direct clinical practice or through the education of nurses. The theorists were risk takers with lifelong commitments to the nursing profession. They viewed nursing as a career rather than as an alternative to marriage, which was the view of many nurses during the 1940s, 1950s, and 1960s. These theorists had broad, well-rounded educational backgrounds and a variety of interests. They were inquisitive, bold, and unafraid to question or challenge the status quo. The demands of their professional lives were great, and their home lives suffered, causing one nursing leader to remark that the early great leaders needed a "wife" to assist them or manage the personal dimension of their lives (R. Schlotfeldt, personal communication with Lisa Eichelberger, 1982). Most of the early theorists made professional choices that affected their personal lives, and most never married or had children. Interestingly, two major universities were responsible for educating most of the early nurse theorists: Peplau, Henderson, Hall, Abdellah, Orlando, Wiedenbach, King, and Rogers all graduated from either Columbia University's Teachers College in New York or Yale University in New Haven, Connecticut.

Why Theories Were Developed

Theory development was an integral part of modern nursing, as evidenced by Nightingale's *Notes on Nursing: What It Is and What It Is Not*, published in 1859. This small book was the first of its kind to theoretically describe the nature of nursing. Research was also an integral part of modern nursing, as evidenced by Nightingale's extensive research projects and publications related to examining the economics and efficacy of army hospitals. Unfortunately, Nightingale's examples of theory development and research were not carried forth. It would be nearly 100 years before nursing theory and research were again considered essential for nurses.

It was not until the 1950s that nurse scholars started to develop *nursing* theories. This occurred during a time when professional thought in nursing was moving toward conceptualizing nursing as a profession based on science rather than as a trade-based apprenticeship. Also at this time, nursing education was in transition, with the education and training of nurses moving into college-level educational institutions and out of hospital-based training schools (Kalisch & Kalisch, 1995).

In the 1960s, the first doctoral programs in nursing were established (Chinn & Kramer, 1999). Prior to the 1960s most nurses who wished to pursue a doctorate did so in related fields such as sociology, education, psychology, and anthropology and then adapted theories from those fields for use in nursing. This approach was initially helpful; however, it became apparent that nursing was unique and contained many aspects not addressed in theories from other disciplines. Other disciplines from which nursing theories were adapted were not immersed in the *actual, real-life particulars* of embodiment; that is, professionally managing the specifics of humans in various states of wellness. For instance, nurses often assess a client's mental, social, and spiritual well-being while at the same time giving a bed bath, evaluating skin integrity, assessing the stage of healing of a surgical wound, and observing for patency of a urinary bladder catheter. Psychologists, sociologists, and anthropologists would generally *not* be expected to provide intimate physical assessment and care while evaluating the psychological and social concerns of an individual or group of individuals. Because of this difference, theories from other related disciplines were (and are) applicable to nursing only in a limited sense. Nursing leaders began to understand that if nursing was to develop its own body of knowledge, the creation of *nursing* theory was essential, and doctoral level *nursing* education and research were critical (Wilde, 1999).

Why the Theorists Created Theories

When the biographies and works of the individual theorists are examined, it becomes apparent that the impetus for developing a theory, model, or framework was two primary reasons: to further nursing as a scholarly profession and to organize and improve the delivery of nursing care. Almost without exception, the nurse theorists created their theories, at least in part, as a result of their direct experiences in practice and their desire to improve practice, whether clinical or classroom based. Imogene King (General Systems Framework) and Martha Rogers (Science of Unitary Human Beings) stated specifically that they developed a conceptual framework/theory because of their concern over the lack of nursing knowledge. These two theorists believed that this knowledge was essential to the development of nursing as a science. Other reasons for theory development given by early theorists were that theories could be tools to provide structure for the improvement of clinical practice, teaching nursing students effectively, or organizing a nursing curriculum.

How Theorists Created Theories

The development of nursing theory started with Nightingale and her astute and mindful observations of actual nursing practice environments. The idea that nursing theory comes from practice is consistent with Dickoff and James's classic theory development article (1968) that says theory about a practice discipline must come from actual practice experience. Discovery of knowledge, concepts, and relationships among and between concepts about the discipline occurs when practitioners are immersed in practice. It is through reflective thinking that practitioners are able to gain insight into the patterns that may exist in the practice arena (Johns, 1994).

Creating a theory is like constructing a complex puzzle (Van Sell & Kalofissudis, 2003). The nurse theorists relate very similar stories as to how they approached theory development. They reflected upon personal and professional experiences to make sense of worldviews and then put together the pieces of the puzzle with the goal of coherent description and explanation.

The nurse theorists used reflection to gain understanding and to glean new knowledge from practice experience. Reflection is an intentional undertaking that requires time and commitment. The purpose of reflection is to allow practitioners to examine clinical anecdotes and resolve contradictions between what the nurse desires to achieve and what is experienced in actual practice, with the goal to achieve more effective outcomes (Johns, 1994). Reflection was described by many of the nurse theorists as one way to generate nursing theory. However, frustration, confusion, the need for organization of content, and the need for a way to communicate outcomes to others also proved helpful in stimulating theory development (Fitne, Inc., 1987–1989).

Theorists wanted to improve the nursing profession and also improve daily clinical nursing care. Reflective practice allowed them to learn and draw conclusions through lived experiences. Nurse theorists sought ways to represent the realities and relationships found within nursing practice. Theories were developed to enhance practice either directly, by stimulating practice-based thinking through reflection, or indirectly, through further development of theory (Ingram, 1991). Said another way, the theorists observed a phenomenon in practice, reflected on it over time, compared it to what was known, and determined goodness of fit and usefulness. Then the phenomenon was named, classified, and categorized, and relationships/interrelationships were described (Peden, 1998).

An example of practice-based theory development can be found in the work of Peplau and her use of participant observation with depressed women (Peplau, 1989). Peplau's work was the earliest published work (1952) after Nightingale. Peplau used several methods of observation, such as interviews, spectator observation, and random observation. She recorded her observations of the nurses and patients, classified and categorized the data, assigned meaning at different levels of abstraction within the phenomenon, and interpreted the observations in the context of the phenomenon. Patterns emerged throughout this process, and Peplau was able to develop interventions from the patterns that helped the patient gain interpersonal competencies during illness (Peden, 1998). It was through this process that Peplau developed her model Interpersonal Relations in Nursing.

Testing of Theory

Theory, practice, and research are interrelated and interdependent. Theory, once conceptualized, must be tested. While theories were being developed in the 1950s and 1960s, doctoral programs in nursing were being established and master's programs were becoming entrenched. Research programs were established, and nurses began to conduct nursing research. Columbia University's Teachers College primarily used a biomedical model for its research focus in the 1950s and concentrated on the roles of nurses. In the 1960s, Yale School of Nursing's research focus was on nursing as a process (George, 2002).

During the subsequent decades, the number and quality of nursing research efforts grew significantly, and the emergence of nursing as a science began. However, there was debate over the methodology being used to study nursing concepts. Since the 1920s, the academic community has primarily used the scientific method of discovery, also known as Logical Positivism, which is based on the assumption that objective truth could be discovered through rigorous observation and experimentation. According to Logical Positivism, a statement or theory is meaningful and adds to knowledge through objective verification: measuring, observing, and quantifying for the purpose of generalizing (Ayers, 1990).

During the late twentieth century, much debate occurred between the social, philosophical, educational, spiritual, and scientific disciplines, and many academic scholars started to view science, theory building, and the generation of knowledge as more of a process rather than as a way to create a "solution" or "discover the truth." The idea of flexibility with regard to the generation of knowledge and theory development started gaining acceptance, and the process of theory development in more recent times has begun to encompass phenomena that cannot be concretely measured and quantified using methods based on the tenets of Logical Positivism (Allmark, 2003). Given the fact that nursing deals with human beings and controlled experimentation is very often impossible, many nurse researchers use qualitative research methods. These qualitative methods, along with alternative approaches, often referred to as "postmodern" methods (Crotty, 1998), are sometimes not fully embraced in the scientific community. Some nurses find these postmodern approaches liberating; others (who still accept Logical Positivism and scientific method as the "gold standard" for knowledge development) are skeptical of these new approaches.

It is normal for individuals to develop opinions that favor one method of theory development and inquiry over another. The kind or type of research one chooses should depend on the questions to be answered rather than on the method of inquiry deemed "acceptable" in most academic circles. Some important questions associated with nursing phenomena that cannot be answered using a controlled, experimental approach lend themselves well to exploration through postmodern methods. An example of such a question might be "What is the experience of parenting a chronically ill child?" Other important nursing questions can be answered only through strict scientific methods of inquiry. An example of this type of question might be "Do axillary temperature measurements in newborns accurately reflect core body temperature?" Approaches spanning Logical Positivism to postmodern methods are essential because of the need for varied tools to use in describing the manifold aspects of nursing practice. All methods contribute to the development of nursing knowledge.

Theory Utilization in Knowledge Development

Nursing theories facilitate the process of describing, explaining, and predicting relevant phenomena, and they support a wide range of research-related endeavors. The best way to truly understand the usefulness of nursing theories is to explore the work of nurses who have utilized them in research studies and other knowledge development activities. The classic, well-established nursing theories presented in this book have formed the theoretical scaffolding upon which many scholarly endeavors have been built and carried out. At the end of each theorist chapter, under the heading "Theory in Action," examples of published knowledge development related to that specific theory are presented.

References

Allmark, P. (2003). Popper and nursing theory. *Nursing Philosophy*, 4(1), 13–16.

Ayers, A. (1990). *Language, truth, and logic* (2nd ed.). London, England: Penguin.

Chinn, P. L., & Kramer, M. K. (1999). *Theory and nursing: Integrated knowledge development*. St. Louis, MO: Mosby.

Crotty, M. (1998). *Foundations of social research: Meaning and perspective in the research process*. London, England: Sage.

Dickoff, J., & James, P. (1968). A theory of theories: A position paper. *Nursing Research,* 17, 197–203.

Fitne, Inc. (Producer). (1987–1989). *Nurse theorists: Portraits of excellence* [DVD]. Available from http://www.fitne.net/nurse_theorists1.jsp

George, J. B. (2002). *Nursing theories: The base for professional nursing practice.* Upper Saddle River, NJ: Prentice Hall.

Ingram, R. (1991). Why does nursing need theory? *Journal of Advanced Nursing,* 16, 350–353.

Johns, C. C. (1994). Guided reflection. In A. Palmer, S. Burns, & C. Bulman (Eds.). *Reflective practice in nursing: Growth of the professional practitioner* (pp. 110–130). Oxford, England: Blackwell Scientific.

Kalisch, P. A., & Kalisch, B. J. (1995). *The advance of American nursing* (3rd ed.). Philadelphia, PA: Lippincott Williams & Wilkins.

Nightingale, F. (1859). *Notes on nursing: What it is, and what it is not.* Philadelphia, PA: Edward Stern and Company.

Peden, A. R. (1998). The evolution of an intervention—the use of Peplau's process of practice-based theory development. *Journal of Psychiatric and Mental Health Nursing,* 5, 173–178.

Peplau, H. E. (1952). *Interpersonal Relations in Nursing.* New York, NY: Putnam.

Peplau, H. E. (1989). Theory: The professional dimension. In A. O. O'Toole & S. Welt (Eds.), *Interpersonal theory in nursing practice: Selected works of Hildegard E. Peplau* (pp. 21–30). New York, NY: Springer.

Van Sell, S. L., & Kalofissudis, I. A. (2003). Formulating nursing theory. Retrieved from http://www.nursing.gr/theory/theory.html

Wilde, M. H. (1999). Why embodiment now? *Advances in Nursing Science,* 22(2), 25–38.

Evaluating a Theory

When evaluating a theory, it is helpful to use a stepwise process, understanding that nursing theories have common components that should be present in some form for others to understand and appreciate the information conveyed. The first step when trying to understand and evaluate a theory is to identify the presence (or absence) of the following six components (Tomey & Alligood, 2002):

1. What concepts are presented that list and classify nursing components of interest?
2. How does the theory define person, health, environment, and nursing?
3. What are the specific statements that clarify exactly what the theory is trying to describe?
4. What types of definitions are used in the theory?
   a. *Theoretical definitions* explain the nature of something in a broad sense and may not be immediately applicable to everyday activities.
   b. *Operational definitions* are meant to explain exactly how something works (e.g., exactly what is meant by "wellness"? What are the observable or measurable signs that a person is experiencing a high degree of wellness?).

5. What are the links or relationships between terms, concepts, and theoretical assertions?

6. How are the concepts and statements organized? (Simple to complex? Linear? Highly structured? Unstructured?)

After forming a basic understanding of what the selected theory is about and identifying the presence or absence of the six components, it is time to evaluate the theory in terms of personal and professional relevance. Consider the following questions based on information found in Chinn and Kramer (1999):

1. What is your gut response to the basic tenets put forth in this theory? Does it make sense in relation to your own professional experience?

2. How clear is this theory? Can you "buy into it"? What factors made this theory either clear or unclear to you (e.g., a feeling or belief that you have held or specificity to a clinical area that you are either familiar or unfamiliar with)?

3. How simple is it? Could you easily describe the overall ideas presented in the theory to a colleague?

4. How general is this theory? Could it be used in many types of nursing settings or is it limited to a selected type of nursing–client situation?

5. How much research exists in current literature that uses this theory as its framework or theoretical base? Choose a time frame (e.g., the years between 1999 and 2003) and conduct a literature search. Is the amount of research using this theory increasing, decreasing, or staying the same?

6. Evaluate the potential impact this theory would most likely have on your current nursing practice. If you used this theory, how significantly would it impact your practice?

Use these steps to gain a basic understanding of each theory presented in this handbook as well as other theories of interest. The point of studying and evaluating a theory is to systematically identify meaningful components, evaluate personal relevance, and then apply new knowledge or understandings where applicable. Continued study and evaluation supports the formation of meaningful insights and opinions that will ultimately deepen professional practice. The most important questions to ask when evaluating theories are:

- Does it resonate with long-held professional insights?
- Does it stimulate new ways of thinking?
- Does it provide fresh viewpoints?

If the answer to any of these questions is "yes," then the theory warrants further exploration.

References

Chinn, P. L., & Kramer, M. K. (1999). *Theory and nursing: Integrated knowledge development.* St. Louis, MO: Mosby.

Tomey, A. M., & Alligood, M. R. (2002). *Nursing theorists and their work* (5th ed.). St. Louis, MO: Mosby.

Theories That Define Nursing or Discuss Nursing in a General Sense: Philosophies

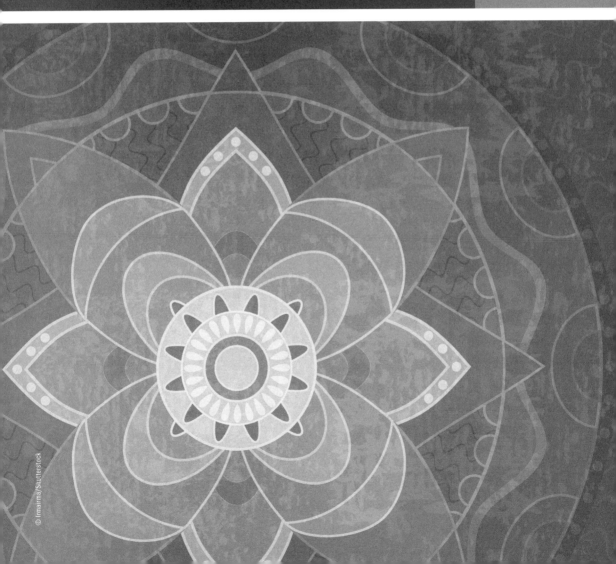

Using the Art of Georges Seurat to Envision Philosophies

The work of some nurse theorists may be classified as *philosophies*. Nursing theories that are classified as philosophies in this text are those created by Nightingale, Henderson, Wiedenbach, and Watson. Philosophies about *nursing in general* seek to define and document what nursing is. A *philosophy* is a system of beliefs regarding the general nature of all things, particularly morality, ethics, and how the world should be viewed. Nursing philosophies address the question "How does nursing fit into the universe?" Nursing practice consists of many realms of activity, so philosophies of *nursing in general* have multiple components that are meant to categorize and clarify the scope and depth of professional activities on a personal and also a global level. The term *professional activities* may include tasks and technical skills, moral/ethical behaviors, personal growth and development, personal knowledge, and professional aesthetic expression (Chinn & Kramer, 1999). Philosophies, therefore, are broad and multidimensional, encompassing both science and art.

Envision the paintings of postimpressionist painter Georges Seurat (1859–1891) when exploring theories that seek to define nursing in general. Seurat perfected a painting technique called pointillism to create vibrant depictions of everyday life in nineteenth-century France. Pointillism is a technique in which tiny points, or dots, of pure color are painstakingly applied to a canvas. The human eye actively "mixes" the colors when viewing the work from a distance of a few feet away or more, thus creating innumerable shades, hues, and depths in the mind's eye. When viewed up close, it is clear that Seurat's works are made up of individual dots, or points, of color. There is beauty in the close-up view because of the brilliance and contrast of each individual dot in relation to the other dots. The play of light on the dots creates the effect of many different shades (see **Color Plate 1** in the color insert).

Perceptions of Seurat's work vary widely among individual viewers and are unique to each person because each "mind's eye" processes the visual input a little differently, especially from a close-up view when only dots of color are perceived. Commonalities of perception become most evident when Seurat's paintings are viewed from far away, when the dots merge into a colorful picture of people, places, and activities. When viewed from a distance, most observers agree that the painting entitled A *Sunday on La Grande Jatte* depicts people out for a stroll in the park (see **Color Plate 2** in the color insert).

In Seurat's works, there is unity and form and, at the same time, a subtle awareness of the interplay between the individual points of color and the larger composition. The color tones may evoke happy, sad, festive, calm, pensive, or other moods. *Bathers at Asnières*, created by Seurat in 1884, evokes calmness and a feeling of contented leisure. The brightness and use of color convey afternoon warmth (see **Color Plate 3** in the color insert).

Seurat's paintings are finite works, with specific themes and bounded visual representations. However, the many points of color within each work seem to merge with the light and color in the surrounding environment to create a feeling of boundlessness.

Theories that explore or describe the phenomenon of nursing in general are similar to Seurat's paintings because each theory is made of distinct points meant to be mixed by the mind's eye so that the viewer may form an impression of nursing as a whole. Most nurses are able to agree on the general concepts presented in theories or descriptions regarding nursing in general, much like those who agree that A *Sunday on La Grande Jatte* depicts people out for a Sunday stroll at the park.

When assessing the many discrete components that make up a general nursing theory or description, individual nurses may have very different impressions about specific meanings because of the unique ways in which the mind processes bits of information, much like differing perceptions of up-close viewers of Seurat's works, wherein the dots of color are processed differently by each person's "mind's eye." Often, disagreements among nurses regarding the content or applicability of a general theory arise from the "close-up" rather than the "faraway" view.

Theories meant to describe or define nursing in a general sense also convey boundlessness, much like the boundlessness evident in Seurat's paintings, in which the light and color in the painting seem to merge with light and color outside the bounds of the canvas. Similarly, in studying general or descriptive theories, one tends to merge personal nursing experiences into the structure of the theory in an attempt to find resonance and meaning, thereby expanding the bounds of the theory into real-life practice. When reading about theories meant to describe nursing in a general sense, assess the information contained in each theory or description from two different vantage points:

- Close-up: What dots of color (ideas) are contained in this theory or description? List the individual ideas (dots of color) that make up the complete picture.
- From a distance: What is the overall composition of this work? What is the "picture," or central idea, that best exemplifies the theory in general? Describe, draw, or obtain a visual representation of it.

Learning Activities

Follow steps one through six to create your own visual images using pointillism (use Color Plate 1 in the color insert as a guide):

1. Gather painting supplies, including watercolor or cardstock-weight paper, acrylic or watercolor paints, and cotton-tipped swabs.
2. Using a pencil, lightly outline simple shapes or other forms on the paper.

3. Using cotton-tipped swabs, dab different colors of paint within and around the shapes previously outlined. Fill each shape with two or three different colors of dots.

4. Experiment with different colors by choosing one or two colors that will appear, or repeat, throughout the picture. Dab several dots of unique color along with several dots of your chosen repeating color(s) inside the drawn shapes until each shape is filled with colors. Keep dabbing until all of the different shapes (and most of the other spaces on the paper) are filled with color.

5. Look at the finished work close-up. Notice how easy it is to differentiate the various dots of color and how challenging it is to discern those basic shapes that were drawn on the paper earlier and each filled with specific combinations of colors.

6. Now look at the finished work from at least 30 feet away. Notice how it becomes difficult to distinguish individual colors and it becomes easier to distinguish those larger basic shapes that were penciled in at the beginning and then filled with specific combinations of colors. (Nursing philosophies are a lot like this. Under close scrutiny, they tend to look like a composition made up of unrelated points with little rhyme or reason; however, when viewed more generally, or from far away, it is easier to discern the gist of the philosophy.)

Reference

Chinn, P. L., & Kramer, M. K. (1999). *Theory and nursing: Integrated knowledge development.* St. Louis, MO: Mosby.

Florence Nightingale's Definition of Nursing

Florence Nightingale (1820–1910) was the second daughter in a wealthy, well-educated, aristocratic English family. Nightingale lived during the Victorian era, an era when upper- and middle-class women were expected to either marry a well-off gentleman or remain with relatives and tend to social and household duties. Nightingale's father highly valued education and provided Nightingale with rigorous tutoring in mathematics, languages, religion, and philosophy. She was a gifted learner and found pleasure and fulfillment in her studies.

Much to the dismay of her family, Nightingale decided that a life of service to humankind was preferable to traditional Victorian marriage or spinsterhood. She completed 3 months of formal nurse training at a Protestant hospital in Germany and then returned to England where she started inspecting and writing about conditions in hospitals, reformatories, and charitable institutions. In 1853, Nightingale became the superintendent of the Hospital for Invalid Gentlewomen in London. In 1854, Nightingale took 38 marginally trained nurses to Scutari, Turkey, during the Crimean War to minister to between 3,000 and 4,000 injured and dying British soldiers wounded in battle. When she first arrived in Scutari, the mortality rate for those admitted to the crude army hospital was 60 percent because of filthy conditions, poor nutrition, and utter despair.

When Nightingale returned to England, the mortality rate stood at just over 1 percent because Nightingale and her nurses dramatically improved hygiene, nutrition, and the level of care to the patients at Scutari. Nightingale became a celebrity in England because of her highly successful efforts in the Crimean War. After returning from the Crimea, Nightingale opened nurse training schools and worked toward the reform of army hospitals. Nightingale used the mathematical skills taught to her by her father to produce statistical analyses of costs and mortality rates associated with running military hospitals.

Through prolific writings, Nightingale expressed the vision that nursing was a vocation and a noble undertaking that required discipline and training. In 1859, Nightingale wrote a slim volume entitled Notes on Nursing: What It Is and What It Is Not. In this book, Nightingale expressed the belief that all women at some time or another would be called upon to "nurse" family or friends, and though "nurses" themselves may or may not have been formally trained, the act of nursing required educated and meticulous planning by those wishing to provide effective nursing care (Nightingale, 1859). Nightingale's slim volume, prolific personal and published writings, as well as the establishment of Nightingale nurse training schools influenced the development of nursing from the Victorian era and into the present time (Kalisch & Kalisch, 1995).

During her lifetime of service and prolific writing, Nightingale did not specifically set out to create a nursing "theory"; however, she did endeavor to define what nursing was. Nightingale discussed many broad moral, spiritual, and personal aspects of what a nurse "should be" in her extant writings, and this is why her published opinions about nursing fall roughly into the category of a philosophy. Just as in the pointillism exhibited in Georges Seurat's paintings, the different points of color (or palette) that might make up Nightingale's rendering of nursing might include the following 10 generalizations:

1. Religious and spiritual beliefs strongly influenced Nightingale's perception of and approach to nursing. For example, the Unitarian faith to which Nightingale belonged strongly supported education [so that God's plan could be fully realized in each human being], so Nightingale focused on the development of nursing education (Montgomery, 2000).

2. Nightingale viewed her involvement in nursing as a higher calling, or vocation, and expressed the belief that other nurses should view the profession in the same way (Kalisch & Kalisch, 1995).

3. Wholism was an early and often-alluded-to concept in Nightingale's writings. For example, she consistently expressed the belief that a nurse should take into account the total environment, client, other persons, the social situation, and any other situationally related factors when providing care (Nightingale, 1859).

4. Nightingale believed that disease in general was a reparative process—nature's (or God's) effort to remedy poisoning, decay, or a reaction against conditions in which a person was placed (Nightingale, 1859).

5. "Nature" and "God" seemed to be synonymous in her writings, indicating the belief of a spiritual foundation for nursing actions based on the natural occurrence of illness (Montgomery, 2000).

6. Nightingale expressed the belief that a nurse's role was to prevent an interruption of the reparative process and to provide optimal conditions for its enhancement through careful observation and committed action to support a calm and reparative environment (Nightingale, 1859).

7. Nightingale believed that nurses should be moral agents and agents of change in society in general (Montgomery, 2000).

8. Another common theme in Nightingale's writing was that nurses should be noble, disciplined, hard-working, and selfless (Nightingale, 1859).

9. Nightingale also expressed the conviction that nurses should be independent decision makers and should provide the physician with precise facts based on sound, educated observations. For example, Nightingale believed that, in order to be effective, those seeking to provide nursing care should receive meticulous education in proper nursing techniques and approaches (Kalisch & Kalisch, 1995).

10. Finally, Nightingale expressed the thought that nursing could (and should) be a means of serving God through selfless service to human-kind and that this selfless service should permeate every aspect of a nurse's existence (Montgomery, 2000).

The finished composition, or "painting," of nursing, consisting of the 10 points of color from the palette just presented might look like this: Nursing is an independent, yet parallel, profession to medicine. Nursing activities should be based on the presumption that all factors within the patient's environment influence healing. Nurses are responsible for recognizing influencing factors and correcting them so that the client's own natural healing ability progresses toward wellness. Nurses should be highly trained and educated to ensure effective care. Nurses must be dignified, of the highest moral fiber, and selfless in the performance of their work. People who choose to become nurses should do so out of a desire to serve God and humanity.

Theory in Action

Nursing theories are meant to stimulate and support knowledge development related to effectively exploring, predicting, describing, defining, and (sometimes) controlling nursing phenomena. Nightingale's work was groundbreaking in that she was the first documented nurse who became an expert statistician to better serve her patients. She set the stage for future nurses to envision themselves as researchers. Through extensive research and writings, both private and published, she significantly influenced healthcare policy in Great Britain. Her influence is still in evidence today, as nurses continue to utilize her work in their own knowledge development activities addressing a variety of issues and concerns. The two publications listed below, which are electronically accessible in the major databases, demonstrate Nightingale's theory in action:

Hegge, M. (2013). Nightingale's environmental theory. *Nursing Science Quarterly*, 26, 211–219. doi:10.1177/0894318413489255

In this article, Hegge describes how she deduced environmental theory from studying Nightingale's work. Throughout her life, Nightingale worked to privately and publicly place focus upon unjust social policies that negatively affected human health. She worked tirelessly to engage the help of policymakers, shape public awareness, and effect positive change for those who were suffering. Nightingale believed that population health should be a priority for nurses.

McDonald, L. (2010). Florence Nightingale: Passionate statistician. *Journal of Holistic Nursing*, 28, 92–98. doi:10.1177/0898010109358769

In this article, McDonald describes how Nightingale's pioneering use and development of statistical methods in relation to health care resulted in significant advances in knowledge development and public policy. Nightingale's work was an expression of her wholistic approach to nursing and her commitment to population health monitoring, advocacy, and positive change.

Learning Activities

Locate and read the two articles listed above to see how nurses have used Nightingale's work.

1. Assess the information contained in Nightingale's theory from two different vantage points:

   - Close-up: What dots of color (ideas) are contained in this theory? List the individual ideas (dots of color) that make up the complete picture.
   - From a distance: What is the overall composition of this work? What is the "picture," or central idea, that best exemplifies the theory in general?

2. Role play: Take turns playing the role of Florence Nightingale and Mary Secole screening women desiring to train as nurses for the Crimean War. The year is 1854. Nightingale and Secole can only ask the recruits five questions each. Decide which five questions they should ask. Use what you learned to help you decide which women will be most suitable to take with you to Crimea. Explain why you think you have chosen the most suitable nurses.

3. Find websites or journal articles about Nightingale and the era in which she lived and worked. Provide the URL, access date, and information about the site host. Words to use when performing a search might include:
   - Florence Nightingale
   - Victorian era
   - Crimean War
   - Nurse training schools
   - Nursing theory

References

Kalisch, P. A., & Kalisch, B. J. (1995). *The advance of American nursing* (3rd ed.). Philadelphia, PA: Lippincott Williams & Wilkins.

Montgomery, B. (2000). *Florence Nightingale: Mystic, visionary, reformer*. Springhouse, PA: Springhouse Publishing.

Nightingale, F. (1859). *Notes on nursing: What it is, and what it is not*. Philadelphia, PA: Edward Stern and Company.

Virginia Henderson's Definition of Nursing

Virginia Henderson (1897–1996) was born the fifth of eight children in Kansas City, Missouri. Because her father's law practice was located in Washington, D.C., the family moved to Virginia, where Henderson spent her childhood. Though her father was an attorney, the family did not have a great deal of money because her father's clients were primarily Native Americans in the western United States and he traveled a great deal (Eichelberger, 1991).

In 1918, Henderson entered the Army School of Nursing in Washington, D.C., and graduated in 1921. Upon graduation, she became a home-visiting community health nurse, working with the Henry Street Settlement in New York City. Henderson stated that her work at the Henry Street Settlement had a significant impact on the development of her views on nursing. In 1922, Henderson began teaching nursing and 5 years later began work on a bachelor's degree and Master of Arts degree in nursing education at Teachers College at Columbia University. In 1930, Henderson became a faculty member at Teachers College and remained there until 1948.

While at Teachers College, Henderson became an author and researcher. Throughout her career she participated in many prestigious writing and research projects. In response to a request from the International Council of Nurses in 1960 to define nursing "independently of technology or medicine" (Henderson, 1960/1997, p. 9), Henderson created a pamphlet entitled *Basic Principles of Nursing Care*. This pamphlet was published by the International Council of Nurses in 1960 and was translated into more than 20 languages.

Henderson never married and spent her retirement years traveling. In 1991, at the age of 93, she traveled to Rome to accept an honorary award before coming before the National League for Nursing to accept yet another national award. Henderson died on March 19, 1996, at the age of 98. The Sigma Theta Tau International Library is named after her, and she left a legacy that will forever be a part of nursing theory history. Henderson has often been called the "First Lady of Nursing."

Because Henderson's definition of nursing is as true today as the day she wrote it, nurses the world over still use her booklet *Basic Principles of Nursing Care*, with the most current revision being in 1997. This small book (or pamphlet, the format in which it was first created) forms the basis of a broad description of nursing; therefore, the general nature of Henderson's work roughly qualifies it as a "nursing philosophy." A quote from the introduction (Henderson, 1960/1997), written by Virginia Henderson, sums up the broad philosophical nature of Henderson's work:

> In this paper, the activities of which basic nursing is composed are outlined. Their origin in universal human needs is stressed and the nurse's continuous interpretation of the way in which these needs are modified by a particular state of the person he or she serves is shown.
>
> The intent is to describe the care that any person requires no matter what the physician's diagnosis and prescribed therapy. . . . The nurse's basic care [approach] is the same whether the patient is considered physically or mentally ill. . . . Because this booklet deals generally with nursing and is applicable to the care of any patient, it can only mention basic nursing activities. (pp. 17–18)

In consideration of the pointillism exhibited in Georges Seurat's paintings, the palette, or points, that might make up Henderson's rendering of nursing include the following (Henderson, 1960/1997, pp. 34–35):

All humans have basic needs that include adequate functioning with respect to:

1. Breathing
2. Eating and drinking
3. Bodily elimination
4. Comfortable body postures
5. Sleeping and resting
6. Selection of proper clothing and maintenance of body temperature and skin integrity
7. Adequate cleanliness
8. Avoiding danger to self and others
9. Communicating meaningfully with others
10. Individually appropriate human developmental tasks
11. Worshipping according to one's faith
12. Work that provides a sense of accomplishment
13. Play and leisure activities
14. Opportunities to learn and satisfy curiosity

Henderson believed that:

> The unique function of the nurse is to assist the individual, sick or well, in the performance of those activities contributing to health or its recovery (or to a peaceful death) that the person would perform unaided given the necessary strength, will or knowledge, and to do this in such a way as to help the individual gain independence as rapidly as possible. (Henderson, 1960/1997, p. 22)

With this defining statement in mind, Henderson identified the components of basic nursing care. These components (more points of color to be added to Henderson's palette) included helping the patient, where needed, with the following (Henderson, 1960/1997, pp. 42–43):

1. Respiration
2. Eating and drinking
3. Elimination
4. Postures and ambulation
5. Sleep and rest requirements
6. Clothing needs

7. Temperature regulation
8. Hygiene
9. Avoiding danger to self and others
10. Communication, especially associated with needs and feelings
11. Religious and spiritual activities
12. The performance of appropriate work activities
13. Play and recreation
14. Learning and human developmental activities

Overall, Henderson expressed the view that a nurse's role is to follow and assist with the medical plan of care outlined by a physician and also to assume the leadership role of planning and providing basic nursing care. Nurses are independent practitioners for providing appropriate basic nursing care; however, they should not independently diagnose an ailment, prescribe medical treatment, or formulate a prognosis. The method by which the nurse facilitates optimal independence for the patient varies from patient to patient and is based on the nurse's professional judgment. Empathy coupled with knowledge and interest on the part of the nurse will enhance the healing process. The overall goal of nursing should be the promotion of as much independence as possible for the patient with regard to Henderson's 14 points.

The finished composition, or "painting," of nursing consisting of the "points of color" (information) provided might look like this: The nurse is an independent practitioner with expertise in aiding the patient to become as independent as possible in life activities. Patient independence is accomplished through appropriate medical intervention that is supported by the nurse and also by excellent basic nursing care that is formulated and carried out by the nurse autonomously. The nurse attends to the wholistic needs of the patient through educated and empathetic attention to the 14 basic needs outlined by Henderson. The nurse is an independent authority on excellent basic nursing care and also a vital aide to other practitioners in the field of health care in ensuring the provision of germane medical treatment for patients with conditions requiring it.

Theory in Action

Nursing theories are meant to stimulate and support knowledge development related to effectively exploring, predicting, describing, defining, and (sometimes) controlling nursing phenomena. Henderson created a basic definition of nursing that clarified basic human needs addressed in nursing care, and nursing's function in assisting patients in meeting those needs. Her work formed a scaffolding upon which many nurses furthered knowledge development through research, writing, and teaching. The two publications listed below, which are electronically accessible through major databases, demonstrate Henderson's theory in action:

Waller-Wise, R. (2013). Utilizing Henderson's nursing theory in childbirth education. *International Journal of Childbirth Education*, 28(2), 30–34. ISSN: 0887-8625

In this article, Waller-Wise utilizes Henderson's 14 Basic Human Needs to create a framework for a childbirth education program in one hospital.

Nicely, B. (2011). Virginia Henderson's principles and practice of nursing applied to organ donation after brain death. *Progress in Transplantation*, 21(1), 72–77. ISSN: 1526-9248

In this article, Nicely utilizes Henderson's Principles and Practice of Nursing in the process of organ donation. Henderson's basic human needs and components of nursing care are applied to the donor's family, friends, and also professional caregivers involved in the process.

Learning Activities

Locate and read the two articles listed above to see how nurses have used Henderson's work.

1. Assess the information contained in this theory from two different vantage points:
   - Close-up: What dots of color (ideas) are contained in this theory? List the individual ideas (dots of color) that make up the complete picture.
   - From a distance: What is the overall composition of this work? What is the "picture," or central idea, that best exemplifies the theory in general?
2. Find a visual representation (photograph, painting, line drawing, sculpture, cartoon), or create one, that expresses Henderson's theory. Glue a copy of the image itself or write a description of the image on a blank sheet to share with your classmates.

3. Find websites or journal articles about Henderson and the era in which she lived and worked. Provide the URL, access date, and information about the site host. Words to use when performing a search might include:
   - Virginia Henderson
   - Virginia Henderson International Library
   - World War I
   - The International Council of Nurses
   - Nursing theory

References

Eichelberger, L. W. (1991). In celebration of Virginia. Retrieved from http://www .clayton.edu/Portals/23/docs/In%20Celebration%20of%20Virginia%20Avenel %20Henderson.doc

Henderson, V. (1997). *Basic principles of nursing care*. Washington, DC: American Nurses Publishing. (Original work published 1960.)

Ernestine Wiedenbach's Helping Art of Clinical Nursing

CHAPTER

8

E rnestine Wiedenbach was born on August 18, 1900, in Hamburg, Germany, to an affluent family. As a young girl of 9 years, Ernestine immigrated with her family to the United States where she became interested in becoming a nurse after observing a private duty nurse take care of her ailing grandmother. Wiedenbach completed a Bachelor of Arts degree at Wellesley College in 1922 and then entered the Johns Hopkins School of Nursing shortly thereafter. After completing her nursing degree at Johns Hopkins in 1925, Wiedenbach worked in many different areas of nursing, including hospital bedside, public health, and administrative nursing. Wiedenbach completed a master's degree and certificate in public health nursing at Teachers College, Columbia University, in 1934. She eventually became a professional nurse writer for the *American Journal of Nursing*. At age 45, Wiedenbach enrolled in the School for Midwives at the Maternity Center Association of New York. After graduating with a degree in midwifery in 1946, Wiedenbach practiced as a nurse midwife and taught evening courses at Teachers College until 1951. Wiedenbach taught at Yale School of Nursing and helped start a master's degree program where she directed the maternal-newborn program. Wiedenbach also continued to publish, writing a textbook in 1958 about family-centered maternity nursing and another in 1964 entitled *Clinical Nursing: A Helping Art*. Wiedenbach retired in 1966 (Tomey & Alligood, 2002).

She is probably most well known for her work in theory development and maternal-child nursing. She never married and died at the age of 97 on March 8, 1998 (Wiedenbach, n.d.).

Wiedenbach asserted that there are four elements to clinical nursing:

1. *Philosophy*: An attitude toward life and reality that evolves from each nurse's beliefs and code of conduct. Philosophy motivates the nurse to act, guides thinking about what to do, and influences decision making (Tomey & Alligood, 2002). According to Wiedenbach, a nursing philosophy has three essential components (George, 2002):
   a. Reverence for the gift of life
   b. Respect for the dignity, worth, autonomy, and individuality of each human being
   c. A resolution to act on personally and professionally held beliefs
2. *Purpose*: That which the nurse wants to accomplish through what he or she does—the overall goals for professional practice, including activities directed toward the overall good of the patient (Tomey & Alligood, 2002).
3. *Practice*: Observable nursing actions that are influenced by disciplined thoughts and feelings toward meeting the patient's need for help. These actions are goal directed and patient centered (Tomey & Alligood, 2002).
4. *Art*: The art of clinical nursing consists of (Tomey & Alligood, 2002):
   a. The nurse's understanding of the patient's condition, situation, and need.
   b. The nurse's internal goals and external actions that are meant to enhance patient capability through appropriate nursing care.
   c. The nurse's activities directed toward improvement of the patient's condition through artful utilization of the medical plan of care.
   d. The nurse's interventions aimed at prevention of recurrence of the current concern or development of a new concern.

Additionally, Wiedenbach further defined her vision of what nursing is in a global sense by defining key terms commonly used to refer to nursing practice. These definitions themselves do not fully define the profession; however, nurses often use global terms such as *patient*, *helping*, *knowledge*, and *nursing action* to loosely describe what they do. In specifically defining what each of these terms means within the context of her theory, Wiedenbach imparts clarity and power to her work and sets the stage for productive exploration and debate.

It may initially seem that definitions for commonly used words or phrases are unnecessary because everyone probably knows what they mean (we are all nurses, right?). However, this is not necessarily the case. Often, such global terms do not mean the same thing to individual nurses or to subgroups within the profession. When two or more nurses discuss nursing within the context of various environments (e.g., when giving and taking report in the hospital, engaging in academic debates or creating written papers in school, or reading and producing published material found in professional journals), they may *think* that they are in total agreement about the meanings of basic terminology when, in fact, they are not. For instance, during a change of shift report, the *reporting* nurse might refer to "excessive stimulus" of a patient and mean to indicate that there were too many relatives in the room visiting all day, whereas the nurse *receiving* the report may construe this to mean that the patient is demonstrating symptoms of internal neurological overstimulation caused by a pathological medical condition. The only way to truly understand what is meant by use of the term *excessive stimulus* is to clarify the definition of the term from the reporting nurse's perspective.

Words are easy to misunderstand, and they are powerful in shaping perceptions, so it is important to carefully define terminology. Here are five terms, defined by Wiedenbach, that elucidate the overall meaning of her theory and clarify what the theory means in terms of actual nursing practice (Tomey & Alligood, 2002):

The *patient* is any person who has entered the healthcare system and is receiving help of some kind, such as care, teaching, or advice. The patient need not be ill; someone receiving health-related education would qualify as a patient.

A *need for help* is defined as any measure desired by the patient that has the potential to restore or extend the patient's ability to cope with various life situations that affect health and wellness.

[Clinical] *judgment* represents the nurse's likeliness to make sound decisions. Sound decisions are based on differentiating fact from assumption and relating them to cause and effect. Sound *judgment* is the result of disciplined functioning of mind and emotions and improves with expanded knowledge and increased clarity of professional purpose.

Nursing *skills* are carried out to achieve a specific patient-centered purpose rather than completion of the skill itself being the end goal. *Skills* are made up of a variety of actions and characterized by harmony of movement, precision, and effective use of self.

Each *person* (whether nurse or patient) is endowed with a unique potential to develop self-sustaining resources. People generally tend toward independence and fulfillment of responsibilities. Self-awareness and self-acceptance are essential to personal integrity and self-worth. Whatever an individual does at any given moment represents the best available judgment for that person at the time.

Wiedenbach describes nursing in a global sense as effective identification of a patient's need for help through observation of presenting behaviors and symptoms, exploration of the *meaning* of those symptoms with the patient, and codetermining the cause(s) of discomfort. The patient's ability to resolve the discomfort is then assessed, and help from the nurse or other healthcare professionals is provided as needed.

The finished composition, or "painting," of nursing consisting of the "points of color" (information) just provided might look like this: Nursing primarily consists of identifying a patient's need for help. If the need for help requires intervention, the nurse facilitates the medical plan of care and also creates and enacts a nursing plan of care based on individual needs and expressed desires of the patient. In providing care, a nurse exercises sound judgment through deliberative, practiced, and educated recognition of sentinel symptoms. The patient's perception of the situation is an important consideration to the nurse when providing competent care. Nurses respect the individuality, dignity, worth, and autonomy of each patient and understand that patients generally value independence. When assessing a patient's need for help and resulting response to care, it is important to remember that human beings generally do the best they can with what they have (emotionally, physically, intellectually, socially), making the best judgments possible *for them* at any given moment. Need for help, and the resulting care provided, is more important than attempting to determine and/or judge *why* a patient may have made a particular life decision.

Theory in Action

Nursing theories are meant to stimulate and support knowledge development related to effectively exploring, predicting, describing, defining, and (sometimes) controlling nursing phenomena. Wiedenbach sought to define clinical nursing and clarify terms commonly used in nursing so that nurses could cultivate commonly held understandings about foundational nursing activities. The three publications listed below, which are electronically accessible in the major databases, demonstrate Wiedenbach's theory in action:

Wiedenbach, E. (1970). Nurses' wisdom in nursing theory. *American Journal of Nursing,* 70(5), 1057–1062.

This sentinel article presents Wiedenbach's assertion that each nurse should identify the theoretical underpinnings that guide personal professional practice in order to better serve patients, families, the profession, and humankind in general. She offers a guide for introspection based on her philosophy of nursing that addresses challenges still evident in nursing today.

Wiedenbach, E. (1951). Safeguard the mother's breasts. *American Journal of Nursing,* 51(9), 544–548.

This historical article addresses the importance of breast care before and after childbirth. Support of the mother and newborn in efforts to breastfeed was stressed. This article was written at a time when formula feeding was the norm, and for this reason, Wiedenbach's work in relation to encouraging breastfeeding was visionary.

Thomas, H., & Wiedenbach, E. (1955). Support during labor. *Hospital Topics,* 33(4), 37–40. doi:10.1080/00185868.1955.9953524

In this article, Thomas and Wiedenbach complete a research study that explores how to appropriately support laboring women. Observation, reflection, and use of a postdelivery questionnaire clarified women's perceptions and preferences during labor and childbirth.

Learning Activities

Locate and read the three articles listed above to learn about application and extension of Wiedenbach's work.

1. Assess the information contained in this theory from two different vantage points:
   - Close-up: What dots of color (ideas) are contained in this theory? List the individual ideas (dots of color) that make up the complete picture.
   - From a distance: What is the overall composition of this work? What is the "picture," or central idea, that best exemplifies the theory in general?
2. Find a visual representation (photograph, painting, line drawing, sculpture, cartoon), or create one, that expresses Wiedenbach's theory. Glue a copy of the image itself or write a description of the image on a blank sheet to share with your classmates.
3. Find websites or journal articles about Wiedenbach and her theory. Words to use when performing a search might include:
   - Ernestine Wiedenbach
   - Nursing theory
   - The Prescriptive Theory of Nursing
   - The Helping Art of Nursing

References

George, J. B. (2002). *Nursing theories: The base for professional nursing practice*. Upper Saddle River, NJ: Prentice Hall.

Tomey, A. M., & Alligood, M. R. (2002). *Nursing theorists and their work* (5th ed.). St. Louis, MO: Mosby.

Weidenbach, E. (n.d.). Ernestine Wiedenbach papers, 1912–1988, MS 1647. Yale University Library. Retrieved from http://drs.library.yale.edu/HLTransformer/ HLTransServlet?stylename=yul.ead2002.xhtml.xsl&pid=mssa:ms.1647& clear-stylesheet-cache=yes

Jean Watson's Theory of Human/Transpersonal Caring

Jean Watson was born in a small, close-knit town in the Appalachian Mountains of West Virginia in the 1940s. Watson graduated from the Lewis Gale School of Nursing in Roanoke, West Virginia, in 1961. After marrying, Watson moved to her husband Doug's home state of Colorado, where she gave birth to two daughters. She continued her nursing studies at the University of Colorado, earning a Bachelor of Science degree in 1964, a Master of Science degree in psychiatric and mental health nursing in 1966, and a doctorate degree in educational psychology and counseling in 1973. Watson then joined the nursing faculty at the University of Colorado Health Sciences Center and served in many teaching and administrative roles, including chair and assistant dean of the undergraduate nursing program, director of the doctoral program, and dean of the School of Nursing. Watson was instrumental in creating the Center for Human Caring at the University of Colorado. This center was created to develop and use knowledge of human caring and healing in nursing and to assist in efforts to transform the healthcare system into a more care-centered entity. Watson lives in Boulder, Colorado, and continues her association with the University of Colorado in the capacity of Distinguished Professor Emerita and Dean Emerita of Nursing. The American Academy of Nursing named Dr. Watson a Living Legend in 2013. Watson founded the Watson Caring Science Institute, a non-profit organization dedicated to transforming and leading healthcare systems in the United States and abroad toward a Caring Science model that values authentic caring-healing relationships grounded in love and compassion (Watson Caring Science Institute and International Caritas Consortium, 2015).

In the following passage, Watson discusses the development of her Theory of Human Caring (Watson, n.d.):

> The Theory of Human Caring was developed between 1975 and 1979, while engaged in teaching at the University of Colorado; it emerged from my own views of nursing, combined and informed by my doctoral studies in educational-clinical and social psychology. It was my initial attempt to bring meaning and focus to nursing as an emerging discipline and distinct health profession with its own unique values, knowledge and practices, with its own ethic and mission to society. The work also was influenced by my involvement with an integrated academic nursing curriculum and efforts to find common meaning and order to nursing that transcended settings, populations, specialty, subspecialty areas, and so forth.
>
> From my emerging perspective, I tried to make explicit nursing's values, knowledge, and practices of human caring that are geared toward subjective inner healing processes and the life world of the experiencing person, requiring unique caring-healing arts and a framework called 10 Caritas Processes™, which complement conventional medicine, and stand in stark contrast to "curative factors." At the same time, this emerging philosophy and theory of human caring seeks to balance the cure orientation of medicine, giving nursing its unique disciplinary, scientific, and professional standing with itself and its public.*

Watson indicates throughout her work that all human beings have an inherent need to participate in caring exchanges, both as giver and receiver, and that nursing holds the essence of this fundamental need.

Because Watson communicates her theory with such clarity, and because the central theme of "care" resonates with so many nurses throughout the world, Watson's Theory of Human/Transpersonal Caring has become a theoretical mainstay for many individual nurses and entire nursing education programs in the United States and around the world.

---

*Theory of Human Caring (retrieved on May 1, 2003, from http://www.uchsc.edu/nursing/caring). Reprinted by permission of Jean Watson.

The major elements that constitute Watson's continually evolving theory are as follows:

- Clinical *caritas* processes (the term *caritas* comes from a Greek term meaning to cherish, appreciate, give special attention to, and value as precious)
- Transpersonal caring relationships
- Caring moments/caring occasions

Other dynamic aspects of the theory that are emerging include the following:

- *Expanded views of self and person* (nurse and client awareness of transpersonal "mindbodyspirit" with unity of being and recognition of embodied spirit)
- *Caring-healing consciousness* (nurse's cultivated intention to care and to promote healing)
- *Caring consciousness* (state of being within the caring exchange mindfully, and recognizing the distinct energy within the caring moment)
- Recognition of the *wholeness and connectedness* of all
- Being open to the belief that a*dvanced caring-healing modalities/nursing arts* constitute a valid future model for the advanced practice of nursing, consciously guided by one's theoretical-philosophical orientation

Here is a closer look at the first major element of Watson's theory, the 10 clinical *caritas* processes. A genuine caring exchange between nurse and client is possible when the nurse mindfully enacts these caring processes (Watson, 2003):

1. Practice of loving-kindness and equanimity within the context of an intentional caring consciousness.
2. Being authentically present.
3. Cultivation of one's own spiritual practices and transpersonal self, going beyond ego self.
4. Developing and sustaining a helping-trusting, authentic caring relationship.

5. Being present to, and supportive of, the expression of positive and negative feelings as a connection with deeper spirit of self and the one being cared for.

6. Creative use of self and all ways of knowing as part of the caring process; to engage in artistry of caring-healing practices.

7. Engaging in genuine teaching-learning experience that attends to unity of being and meaning, while attempting to stay within other's frame of reference.

8. Creating a healing environment at all levels (physical as well as non-physical, subtle environment of energy and consciousness), whereby wholeness, beauty, comfort, dignity, and peace are potentiated.

9. Assisting with basic needs, with an intentional caring consciousness, administering human care essentials, which potentiate alignment of mindbodyspirit, wholeness, and unity of being in all aspects of care; tending to both embodied spirit and evolving spiritual emergence of both other and self.

10. Opening and attending to spiritual-mysterious and existential dimensions of one's own life–death; soul care for self and the one being cared for.

These 10 caring processes outline a nursing practice whereby it is recognized by the nurse that all of life is interconnected. Each nurse–client exchange is made up of shared energy among all who are present during the interaction. The nurse is called not only to recognize the evolving physical/spiritual being in the client being cared for but also to recognize and nurture the physical/spiritual being in the self, for one cannot provide authentic caring to another without first being able to care for the self.

The second major element of Watson's theory is *transpersonal caring relationship*. Transpersonal caring relationships are the foundation of nursing work. Transpersonal caring seeks to connect with and embrace the spirit or soul of the other through the processes of caring and healing and being in authentic relation, in the moment (Watson, 2003). Transpersonal caring implies that the nurse consciously focuses on the uniqueness of self, other, and the present moment, wherein the nurse–client exchange is mutual and reciprocal, each fully embodied in the moment, while paradoxically capable of transcending the moment and opening to new possibilities. Transpersonal caring calls for personal reflection and an ability on the part of the nurse to be mindfully present to self and others. The transpersonal nurse has the ability to center consciousness and intentionality on caring, healing, and wholeness rather than on disease, illness, and pathology. The nurse attempts to enter into and stay within the other's frame of reference for connecting with the inner life world of meaning and spirit of the other. Together they join in a mutual search for meaning and wholeness. The authentic transpersonal caring exchange will potentiate comfort measures, pain control, a sense of well-being, wholeness, and/or even spiritual transcendence of suffering. The person is viewed as whole and complete, regardless of illness or disease (Watson, 2003).

The third major element of Watson's theory is *caring moments/caring occasions*. A caring occasion occurs whenever the nurse and patient come together with their unique life histories and phenomenal fields in a human-to-human transaction. The coming together in a given moment becomes a focal point in space and time. It becomes transcendent, whereby experience and perception take place, but the actual caring occasion has a greater field of its own in a given moment. The process goes beyond itself, yet arises from aspects of itself that become part of the life history of each person, as well as part of some larger, more complex pattern of life (Watson, 1988). A caring moment consists of actions and choices made by both the nurse and the patient. The moment of coming together presents each with the opportunity to decide how to participate in the relationship. If the caring moment is transpersonal, the client and nurse feel connected with one another at the spiritual level, and thus the moments in the interaction transcend time and space and open up new possibilities for healing and human connection at a deeper level than physical, social, or verbal interaction (Watson, 2003).

In summary, Watson's theory is about mindful, in-the-moment, committed caring for both self and patient. One of the rewards of enacting Watson's theory in daily nursing practice is deeper knowledge, understanding of, and compassion for self and others. Watson writes:

> We learn from one another how to be human by identifying ourselves
> with others, [and] finding their dilemmas in ourselves. What we all
> learn from it is self-knowledge. The self we learn about . . . is every
> self. IT is universal—the human self. We learn to recognize ourselves in
> others. . . . [This kind of interaction] keeps alive our common humanity
> and avoids reducing self or other to the moral status of object.
> (Watson & Ray, 1988, pp. 59–60)

The finished composition, or "painting," of nursing, consisting of the "points of color" from the palette of information contained in Watson's theory might look like this: Nursing primarily consists of a core of intentional caring intertwined with excellent nursing skills. The nurse and patient are equally valued in the nurse–patient interaction, with both contributing various attributes to the caring environment. Central to excellent transpersonal caring on the part of the nurse is the realization that connections between patient and nurse exist on many levels, from the overt physical environment to deep levels of energy exchange that are not readily observable in the traditional sense. Spirituality, intentionality, and mindful attention to the here and now within the human-to-human exchange enables the nurse to wholistically express caring in the physical, emotional, psychological, spiritual, social, and matter/energy realms simultaneously.

Envision rainbows of light particles surrounding and enveloping the nurse and patient. These particles are vibrating, intermingling, ebbing, and flowing as the transpersonal moment occurs. At close proximity, individual colors emitted by both the patient and the nurse intensify and mix, and when the two move away from each other the colors soften and become pale. When nurse and patient conclude the interaction, and one or the other moves increasingly away, there is a pale trail of vibrating color that follows each participant, with lingering hues of the nurse within the client and the client within the nurse.

Jean Watson: Personal Experience and Background in Being a Nurse Theorist

One never expects, or at least I never expected, nor anticipated, being a so-called nurse theorist. It happened gradually and indirectly, along the way, via a process of scholarly writing in my efforts to make sense of nursing. My journey began as a process of exploring deep meaning, integrity, distinction, and philosophical underpinning of the nature of nursing. This exploration was influenced by having a background in psychiatric mental health nursing and having completed my PhD, studying various existential and phenomenological aspects of human existence. These experiences allowed me the privilege of examining the diverse theories or personality, ways of being in the world, and exploring various views of humanity, dynamics of human behavior, and so on.

Writing my first book was also a healing experience for me personally, in that I had just joined the faculty of the University of Colorado and was distressed that most of the focus and direction for advancing nursing was within the context of medical science, technology, and conventional research related to disease treatment and curing, almost at all costs.

Thus, after completing my PhD and drawing upon my intellectual and educational clinical experiences and my master's degree in psychiatric-mental health nursing, my journey began more formally. My first book, *Nursing: The Philosophy and Science of Caring* (1979, 1985), was triggered by my new academic world entry and critique of status quo with medical focus on nursing. It began my exploration of core values, knowledge, and context for nursing science, with its focus on humanity and human caring, healing, human experiences, and health in contrast with, but complementary to medical science. It offered a philosophical and scientific-research orientation, as well as a language and structure for the phenomenon of human caring.

In this first work, I was asking myself the question, "Is there a core of nursing that transcends medical cure approaches and clinical settings, diagnoses, treatments, and so on that relates to what nursing offers to humanity?" Further, I was questioning whether there is a core of nursing that is universal and timeless that is not defined by tasks and skills and actions that nurses do, while pursuing a framework of human caring that defines nursing and its contribution to society, beyond medicine and medical science.

That same personal exploratory process of mine acknowledged that the current state of nursing was void of a meaningful philosophical foundation for its model of science. Therefore, my first book offered a personal answer to my own quest/questioning and served as a treatise and guide for defining and advancing nursing for its future, while honoring, identifying, and naming nurses and nursing's timeless and ancient gift to humankind. Further, I wanted to acknowledge to nursing and the public the essential nature of nursing's role in human caring, health, and well-being, which needs to be sustained and advanced if human caring is to evolve and survive in the world. It was a decade or so later that my work began to be considered a theory and be discovered as a meaningful philosophical-theoretical framework for nursing.

Personal Views of Being a Nurse Theorist

On a more personal level, especially because my work has been studied and explored via professional practice models, empirical validation through research, and educational curricular models, I have received offers of remarkable learning experiences around the world. My studies and contact with students, faculty, and clinicians have included every continent; I have been around the world at least 12 times, touching the hearts and lives and minds of nurses in hospitals, educational programs, and diverse clinical settings.

Likewise, these many thousands of nurses have expanded and deeply touched my mind, heart, and life by helping to affirm and extend my own thinking and scholarship. My latest work has evolved as a model of caring science, which provides a framework both for nursing and beyond nursing, allowing diverse theories to be explored and located within a shared worldview. Caring science unites and seeks converging ideas and models, within a unitary worldview and ethic of belonging to an infinite field of universal love, which holds the world and humanity in a global field (Levinas, 1969; Watson, 2005).

My work also requires personal practices of my own theory in order to sustain authenticity and dynamic evolution, constantly changing toward more depth and wisdom, beyond knowledge per se. Thus, my first *caritas* process, *cultivation of loving kindness and equanimity toward self and other*, requires my engagement as well as acknowledging such basic practices for self, in order to sustain humanistic altruistic values and authentic caring presence and relationship with others. Thus, I still am trying to catch up with my own theory, because it is larger and deeper than my own knowledge, but an ongoing personal, spiritual journey toward inner life world of self, honoring the deep subjective inner life world of self/other. This personal/professional practice seeks to "see" who is the spirit-filled person behind the physical appearance, behind the diagnosis and treatment, behind the behavior I/we may not like or approve. This reminds me and others that one person's level of humanity reflects on the other, and therefore, caring theory is an ongoing dynamic process of understanding life and all the vicissitudes of human existence, from birth to death and beyond— seeking wisdom, compassion, love, and personal integration of knowledge and all of life's known and unknown experiences. This work embraces mystery, humility, and surrender, while trusting in deep love and one's soul journey on the Earth plane.

Other Personal Notes

My life experiences and own personal tragedies/blessings have been my teachers and also influenced my writings and theory expansions. For example, having a serious traumatic eye injury several years ago allowed me the gift of receiving and experiencing my own theory of caring from my husband. I had to be still for almost 3 months, with only 15-minute breaks, lying face down on a massage table, allowing for the eye to heal. This time of stillness and quiet contemplation awakened a deeper appreciation of life and all the small things we take for granted. Further, my own theory guided my approach to my care. Rituals, beauty, nature, meditation, music/sound, silence, and intentional loving touch therapies and massage were incorporated into my caring. No negative energy, such as television or newspapers, was allowed into my healing space; people took off their shoes when they entered the room. Poetry and literature and healing cards were read to me. I was given full body massages; I dwelled in silence and contemplative time for meditation. I was grateful for everything and life itself; I treasured listening to sounds of nature and using a mirror to look outside my window, even upside down, to see the trees, sky, and birds. I wrote psalms as a meditative and sacred act of expression and release (Watson, 1999).

I cherished basic daily living activities and engaged in meditation and praying without ceasing, as a way to sustain myself and my emotional, psychic, and physical pain. All of these experiences, painful and otherwise, both validated and affirmed my theory of caring and healing, while allowing me the privilege of experiencing it from the inside out. These and other experiences provided more personal/professional confidence and courage related to my philosophies and theory, leading to my book, *Caring Science as Sacred Science* (2005). This book acknowledged the sacredness of all of nursing, in that we are dealing with the life force and mystery of life itself.

Other personal practices that continue to inform my work and writings include exposure to nurses in many other cultures; these global cultural human experiences help me to appreciate and deepen my understanding of the universality of human conditions and the timeless need for human caring and healing. Such knowledge, wisdom, and insights go beyond conventional medical-scientific approaches that often restrict nurses in their education and practices and learning of human caring, healing, and health.

More recently I am blessed to be working with many hospitals, nurses, and other staff to deepen and sustain human caring theory as a living intellectual model of authentic heart-centered practices of *caritas* nursing and health care—restoring love and caring as the foundation for healing self and other, thus transforming self and systems. Such experiments and pilot programs are seeking criteria to designate hospitals as authentic caring science institutions, not confined to medical-techno-cure focus, rather returning to caring and love as the core of healing and healing environments. Thus, my personal professional journey continues to intersect, as the personal becomes the professional, in a living model of caring science.

Most recently my work is culminating and continuing through Watson Caring Science Institute, a nonprofit foundation, created in 2007 to extend and deepen caring science work in the world. The foundation's website is at www.watsoncaringscience.org. The latest project is acknowledging to the public that nurses and nursing stand as an archetype for human caring and love to humanity. This project is designed to reach a million nurses, meditating at the same time, to radiate a global caring field to humanity around the world; this project coincides with the international year of the nurse in 2010. The global caring field meditation project began January 1, 2010, at noon, wherever anyone was in the world. The global caring field meditation is scheduled to be repeated on May 12, 2010, which is Florence Nightingale's birthday and her centenary year. It concludes on December 31, 2010, yet extends into 2011 with the Hiroshima International Conference on Caring and Peace, making new connections between the nurse's role in sustaining human caring and affirming the relationship between caring and peace in the world.

Finally, the work in caring science allows for a full maturation of nursing as a distinct discipline and profession in its own right, offering wisdom, vision, and sustaining directions for the future of caring and healing for humanity, and its evolution toward a moral community of global caring, healing, and health for all.

Key Background Representative Books

Bevis, E. O., & Watson, J. (1989). *Toward a caring curriculum: A new pedagogy for nursing.* New York: National League for Nursing.

Bevis, E. O., & Watson, J. (2000). *Toward a caring curriculum. A new pedagogy for nursing.* Sudbury, MA: Jones and Bartlett.

Chinn, P., & Watson, J. (Eds.). (1994). *Art and aesthetics of nursing*. New York, NY: National League for Nursing.

Leininger, M., & Watson, J. (Eds.). (1990). *The caring imperative in education*. New York, NY: National League for Nursing.

Levinas, E. (1969). *Totality and infinity: An essay on exteriority*. Pittsburgh, PA: Duquesne University Press.

Sitzman, K., & Watson, J. (2014). *Caring science, mindful practice: Implementing Watson's human caring theory*. New York, NY: Springer.

Taylor, R., & Watson, J. (Eds.). (1989). *They shall not hurt: Human suffering and human caring*. Boulder, CO: University Press of Colorado.

Watson, J. (Ed.). (1994). *Applying the art and science of human caring*. New York, NY: National League for Nursing.

Watson, J. (1999). *Nursing: Human science and human care* (3rd ed.). New York, NY: Appleton-Century-Crofts.

Watson, J. (1999). *Postmodern nursing and beyond*. Edinburgh, Scotland, UK: Churchill Livingstone/W. B. Saunders.

Watson, J. (2002). *Assessing and measuring caring in nursing and health sciences*. New York, NY: Springer.

Watson, J. (2005). *Caring science as sacred science*. Philadelphia, PA: F. A. Davis Company.

Watson, J. (2007). Reconsidering nursing education scholarship. In U. Zeitler (Ed.), *Center for innovation in nursing education*. Aarhus, Denmark: The Center for Innovation in Nursing Education.

Watson, J. (2008). *Assessing and measuring caring in nursing and health sciences* (2nd rev. ed.). New York, NY: Springer.

Watson, J. (2008). *Nursing: The philosophy and science of caring* (Revised and updated ed.). Boulder: University Press of Colorado.

Watson, J., & Ray, M. (Eds.). (1988). *The ethics of care and the ethics of cure: Synthesis in chronicity*. New York, NY: National League for Nursing.

Key Background Representative Journal Articles

(* = Refereed journal)

*Cowling, R., Smith, M., Watson, J., & Newman, M. (2008). The power of wholeness, consciousness, and caring. A dialogue on nursing science, art and healing. *Advances in Nursing Science*, 31(1), E41–E51.

*Fawcett, J. (2002). The nurse theorists: 21st century updates—Jean Watson. *Nursing Science Quarterly*, 15(3), 214–219.

*Fawcett, J., Watson, J., Neuman, B., & Hinton-Walker, P. (2001). On theories and evidence. *Journal of Nursing Scholarship*, 33(2), 121–128.

*Foster, R. (contributor). (2007). Tribute to the theorists: Jean Watson over the years. *Nursing Science Quarterly*, 20(1), 7.

*Hemsley, M. S., Glass, N., & Watson, J. (2006). Taking the eagle's view: Using Watson's conceptual model to investigate the extraordinary and transformative experiences of nurse healers. *Journal of Holistic Nursing Practice*, 20(2), 85–94.

*Johns, C., & Watson, J. (Eds.). (1999). Reflective caring practices [Guest editorial]. *International Journal of Human Caring*, 3(2), 5–7.

*Persky, G., Nelson, J. W., Watson, J., & Bent, K. (2008). Profile of a nurse effective in caring. *Nursing Administration Quarterly*, 32(1), 15–20.

*Quinn, J. F., Smith, M., Ritenbaugh, C., Swanson, K., & Watson, M. J. (2003). Research guidelines for assessing the impact of the healing relationship in clinical nursing. *Alternative Therapies in Health and Medicine*, 9(Suppl. 3), A65–A79.

*Watson, J. (1998). Nightingale and the enduring legacy of transpersonal human caring. *Journal of Holistic Nursing*, 16(2), 292–294.

*Watson, J. (2000). Leading via caring-healing: The four-fold way toward transformative leadership. *Nursing Administration Quarterly*, 25(1), 1–6.

*Watson, J. (2000). Postmodern nursing: Revisioning nursing's transpersonal caring. *Hong Kong Nursing Journal*, 36(4), 31–33.

*Watson, J. (2000). Reconsidering caring in the home. *Journal of Geriatric Nursing*, 21(6), 330–331.

*Watson, J. (2000). Via negativa: Considering caring by way of non-caring. *Australian Journal of Holistic Nursing*, 7(1), 4–8.

*Watson, J. (2001). Post-hospital nursing: Shortages, shifts, and scripts. *Nursing Administrative Quarterly*, 25(3), 77–82.

*Watson, J. (2002). Caring and healing our living and dying. *International Nurse*, 15(2), 4–5.

*Watson, J. (2002). Holistic nursing and caring: A values based approach. *Journal of Japan Academy of Nursing Science*, 22(2), 69–74.

*Watson, J. (2002). Intentionality and caring-healing consciousness: A theory of transpersonal nursing. *Holistic Nursing Practice*, 16(4), 12–19.

*Watson, J. (2002). Metaphysics of virtual caring communities. *International Journal of Human Caring*, 6(1), 41–45.

*Watson, J. (2002, Spring). Nursing: Seeking its source and survival [Guest editorial]. *ICUs and Nursing Web Journal*, 9, 1–7. Retrieved from http://watsoncaringscience .org/files/PDF/WatsonICU02.pdf

*Watson, J. (2003). Love and caring: Ethics of face and hand. *Nursing Administration Quarterly*, 27(3), 197–202.

*Watson, J. (2004). *Caritas* and *communitas*: An ethic for caring science. *Journal Japan Academy of Nursing Science*, 24(1), 66–71.

*Watson, J. (2004). The relational core of nursing as partnership [Invited commentary]. *Journal of Advanced Nursing*, 47(3), 241–250.

*Watson, J. (2005). Caring science: Belonging before being as ethical cosmology. *Nursing Science Quarterly*, 18(4), 4–5.

*Watson, J. (2005). Commentary on Shattell, M. (2004). Nurse-patient interaction: A review of the literature. *Journal of Clinical Nursing*, 14, 530–532.

*Watson, J. (2005). Current issues and haunting concerns for survival of nursing profession. *Japanese Journal of Nursing Science*, 30(11), 50–53.

Watson, J. (2005). Love and caring [Reposted]. *Alternative Journal of Nursing*, 9. Retrieved from http://www.altjn.com/perspectives/love_caring.pdf

Watson, J. (2005). An overview of Watson's theory of human caring. *Bulletin of Japanese Red Cross University College of Nursing*, 19, 2005.

*Watson, J. (2005). What, may I ask, is happening to nursing knowledge and professional practices? What is nursing thinking at this turn in human history? [Editorial]. *Journal of Clinical Nursing*, 14, 913–914.

*Watson, J. (2006). Can an ethic of caring be maintained? *Journal of Advanced Nursing*, 54(3), 257–259.

*Watson, J. (2006). Carative factors—*Caritas* processes guide to professional nursing. *Danish Clinical Nursing Journal*, 20(3), 21–27.

*Watson, J. (2006). Caring theory as ethical guide to administrative and clinical practices. *Nursing Administrative Quarterly*, 30(1), 48–55.

Watson, J. (2006). Caring theory as ethical guide to administrative and clinical practices. *JONA'S Healthcare Law, Ethics, and Regulation*, 8(1), 87–83.

*Watson, J. (2006). Frontline and backstage caring: American nurse/world-wide nurses. *American Nurse Today*, 1(1), 24–28.

*Watson, J. (2006). Spiritual pilgrimage as *caritas* action in the world. *Journal of Holistic Nursing*, 24(4), 289–296.

*Watson, J. (2007). Theoretical questions and concerns: Responses from a caring science framework. *Nursing Science Quarterly*, 20(1), 13–15.

*Watson, J. (2007). Watson's theory of human caring and subjective living experiences: Disciplinary guide to professional nursing practice. *Brazilian Clinical Nursing Journal: Texto and Contexto*, 16(1), 129–135.

*Watson, J. (2008). Social justice and caring: A model of caring science as a hopeful paradigm for moral justice for humanity. *Creative Nursing: A Journal of Values, Issues, Experience & Collaboration*, 14(22), 54–61.

*Watson, J. (2009). Caring science and human caring theory: Transforming personal/professional practices in nursing and healthcare. *Journal of Health and Human Services Administration*, 31(4, symposium issue), 466–482.

*Watson, J. (2009). Concept of caring from Watson's perspective. *Nursing Science Quarterly*, 22(3).

*Watson, J. (2009). From theory to practice: Caring science according to Watson and Brewer. *Nursing Science Quarterly*, 22(4), 339–345.

*Watson, J., Bauer, R., & Biley, F. (2002). Bavarian nursing secret: An inside view. *Reflections on Nursing Leadership: Sigma Theta Tau International Magazine*, 28(1), 26–28.

*Watson, J., Biley, F. C., & Biley, A. M. (2002). Aesthetics, postmodern nursing, complementary therapies and more: An Internet dialogue. *Complementary Therapies in Nursing and Midwifery*, 8, 81–83.

*Watson, J., & Foster, R. (2003). The attending nurse caring model: Integrating theory, evidence and advanced caring-healing therapeutics for transforming professional practice. *Journal of Clinical Nursing*, 12, 360–365.

Watson, J., & Smith, M. C. (2002). Caring science and the science of unitary human beings: A trans-theoretical discourse for nursing knowledge development. *Journal of Advanced Nursing*, 37(5), 452–461.

Theory in Action

Nursing theories are meant to stimulate and support knowledge development related to effectively exploring, predicting, describing, defining, and (sometimes) controlling nursing phenomena. Watson's work related to establishing deep caring comportment as the foundation of nursing care has stimulated extensive knowledge development. The three publications listed below, which are electronically accessible in the major databases, demonstrate Watson's theory in action:

Arslan-Ozkan, I., Okumus, H., & Buldukoglu, K. (2013). A randomized controlled trial of the effects of nursing care based on Watson's Theory of Human Caring on distress, self-efficacy and adjustment in infertile women. *Journal of Advanced Nursing*, 70(8), 1801–1812.

This article details a research study that explored the effects of caritas nursing in situations where women were experiencing the challenges of infertility.

Piccinato, J. M., & Rosenbaum, J. N. (1997). Caregiver hardiness explored within Watson's Theory of Human Caring in nursing. *Journal of Gerontological Nursing*, 23(10), 32–39.

In this analytical article, the authors explore the theoretical concept of caregiver hardiness through the lens of Watson's theory.

Sitzman, K. (2010). Student-preferred caring behaviors for online nursing education. *Nursing Education Perspectives*, 31(3), 171–178.

This research study was built upon the theoretical foundation of Watson's Theory of Human Caring. It utilized a survey format to identify nursing instructor behaviors that convey and sustain caring in online classrooms.

Learning Activities

Locate and read the three articles listed above to see how nurses have used Watson's work.

1. Assess the information contained in this theory from two different vantage points:
    *   Close-up: What dots of color (ideas) are contained in this theory? List the individual ideas (dots of color) that make up the complete picture.

- From a distance: What is the overall composition of this work? What is the "picture," or central idea, that best exemplifies the theory in general?

2. Find a visual representation (photograph, painting, line drawing, sculpture, cartoon), or create one, that expresses Watson's theory. Glue a copy of the image itself or write a description of the image on a blank sheet to share with your classmates.

3. Find websites about Watson's theory or locate journal articles about her life and theories. Words to use when performing a search might include:
   - Jean Watson
   - Theory of Human Caring
   - Nursing theory
   - Alternative therapies

4. Compare and contrast the similarities and differences among the four nurses who have given us the nursing philosophies described in Part II. How are they alike personally, professionally, conceptually, and ideally? How are they different? What makes each unique? What part do you think their differences played in the development of each unique nursing philosophy?

5. If you could ask any one of the four theorists discussed in Part II one question, which theorist would you ask, what would you ask them, and why would you want to know?

References

Levinas, E. (1969). *Totality and infinity: An essay on exteriority*. Pittsburgh, PA: Duquesne University Press.

Watson, J. (n.d.). *Theory of Human Caring*. Retrieved from http://watsoncaringscience.org/images/features/library/THEORY%20OF%20HUMAN%20CARING_Website.pdf

Watson, J. (1988). New dimensions of human caring theory. *Nursing Science Quarterly*, 1(4), 175–181.

Watson, J. (2003). Ten caritas processes. Retrieved from http://watsoncaringscience.org/about-us/caring-science-definitions-processes-theory/global-translations-10-caritas-processes/

Watson, J. (2005). *Caring science as sacred science*. Philadelphia, PA: F. A. Davis Company.

Watson Caring Science Institute and International Caritas Consortium. (2015). WCSI fact sheet. Retrieved from http://watsoncaringscience.org/about-us/wcsi-fact-sheet/

Watson, J., & Ray, M. (Eds.). (1988). *The ethics of care and the ethics of cure: Synthesis in chronicity*. New York, NY: National League for Nursing.

Theories About Broad Nursing Practice Areas: Grand Theories

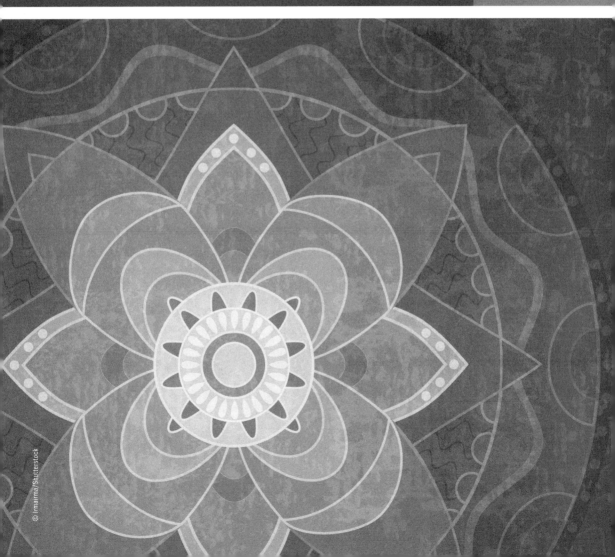

Envisioning Theories Through Mandala Art

The purpose of a *grand theory* is to organize various pieces of information around an identified broad concept, or central point, associated with nursing practice. This is done so that other nurses may better understand the individual components that influence nursing perceptions and practices connected to a specific concept. For example, nurses routinely discuss issues surrounding "health" and "wellness" when providing care in a wide range of settings. Different nurses may have dissimilar perceptions about what factors influence or determine states of "health" and "wellness." These differences may dramatically affect how nursing care is delivered by individual nurses; thus, it becomes useful to formally explore and clarify the terms *health* and *wellness* so that nurses, as a group, may productively use, discuss, and investigate these important concepts.

In art, mandalas are forms in which there is a central, or focal, point around which multiple symmetrically arranged elements exist. In mandalas, an infinite number of patterns may be formed around an infinite number of unique focal points. Mandalas are abundant in nature, appearing, for example, in human cells, snowflakes, flowers, the iris of the eye, spider webs, whirlpools, and tornadoes. All have a center point around which multiple elements are arranged, creating unity and completeness. Throughout history, human beings in all cultures have recognized mandalas in nature and have sought to create their own mandalas to visually represent uniquely human interests. Even today, this ancient art form has many enthusiasts, as evidenced by the existence of numerous mandala artists, books, clubs, and websites, which are accessed by thousands of people around the world every day. **Color Plate 5**, found in the color insert section of this text, shows an image from a website where people share personal mandala art creations.

Here are other representations of mandalas used around the world:

- Many Christian cathedrals in Europe have labyrinths. Labyrinths are similar to mandalas in that they have a central point around which symmetrically arranged elements form a balanced pattern, in some form or another, on the floors, walls, and ceilings. Many believe that walking a labyrinth, or tracing the outline of a smaller one with a finger or stylus, induces a calm, meditative state wherein the order, unity, and beauty of the universe may be contemplated. Amiens Cathedral in France was completed around 1289. This cathedral has a tile labyrinth on the floor (**Color Plate 6**) on which hundreds of visitors a year contemplatively walk the lines that form the design (**Color Plate 7**).
- Mandalas can be seen in most Christian cathedrals all over the world in the form of rose windows (**Color Plate 8**) or other decorative designs such as the one found in the bottom of a baptismal font (**Color Plate 9**). Both photos are from the Cathedral of the Madeleine in Salt Lake City, Utah.
- In the Buddhist tradition, intricate sand mandalas are created, viewed for a short time, and then swept away to represent the cycle of life and rebirth and to represent the impermanence of all things. The sand mandala shown in **Color Plate 10** was created in June 2003 at the Philadelphia Museum of Art by the Venerable Losang Samten.
- The mandala form is also evident in English, Asian, and Greek gardens, as evidenced by a contemporary garden in Canada (**Color Plate 11**).

Mandalas are useful in illustrating the concept of *grand theories* in nursing because, like grand theories, mandalas contain a central point of interest surrounded by smaller components organized into a unified work. Like grand theories, mandalas are purposely arranged to provide beauty and clarity. Both have distinct boundaries meant to provide a sense of unity and completeness; however, the symmetry of the design easily allows for the inclusion of additional layers without significantly altering the central point.

When reading about theories that contain a broad, central point of interest, systematically surrounded by supporting or explanatory concepts, envision a mandala and ask these 10 questions:

1. What is the central point around which all of the smaller concepts cluster?
2. What are the names of the smaller concepts?
3. Where do the smaller concepts fall in relation to the central concept?
4. Envision whether a smaller concept is closely related to the central concept, thereby belonging close to the center of the design, or whether it is a more loosely connected concept that would belong on the periphery of the design.
5. Would the central concept be large, occupying most of the space in the overall design, or small, with the supporting components occupying most of the space?
6. Are there many small components of equal size, or are there some components that are significantly larger than others?
7. Would the theory form a smooth, circular design, or a linear, angular design?
8. Would the completed design appear cluttered or sparse with regard to number, size, and spacing of central and peripheral elements?
9. Would the peripheral margins of the design be open or closed?
10. What colors would you choose to use in each component of the design?

With mandala art, it is important to experience the creation (or completion through coloring) of a design. Through kinesthetic and nonverbal learning pathways, as accomplished through coloring, it is possible to deepen one's understanding of these rich and powerful art forms and to get a better feel for how they apply to grand theory structure. Color the mandala in **Figure 10.1** with crayons, colored pencils, or paints. Focus on the center and contemplate how the rest of the design symmetrically grows outward. This design has many components; however, the overall effect is one of unity and completeness. While coloring, be mindful of how the components are distinct, yet connected. When the project is complete, close the book and avoid viewing it for several hours or more. When viewed later with a fresh eye, a mandala may appear more unified and hold meanings that were not apparent during the creative process of completing it.

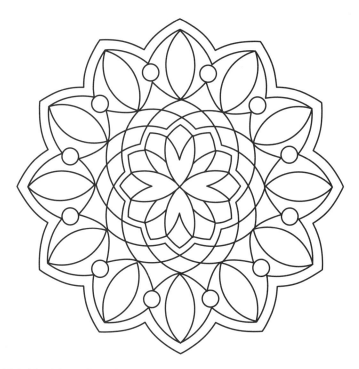

Figure 10.1 Mandala art form. Reprinted with permission from a mandala coloring book created by Monique Mandali. To view more mandalas or to order a mandala coloring book, go to www.mandali.com.
Courtesy of http://www.mandali.com.

Myra Estrin Levine's Conservation Model

Myra Estrin Levine (1920–1976) was born in Chicago, Illinois. She was the oldest of three children. Levine developed an interest in nursing because her father was frequently ill and required nursing care on many occasions. Levine graduated from the Cook County School of Nursing in 1944 and obtained her Bachelor of Science degree in nursing from the University of Chicago in 1949. Following graduation, Levine worked as a private duty nurse, as a civilian nurse for the U.S. Army, as a surgical nursing supervisor, and in nursing administration. After earning a Master of Science degree in nursing at Wayne State University in 1962, she taught nursing at many different institutions (George, 2002).

Levine told others that she did not set out to develop a "nursing theory" but had wanted to find a way to teach the major concepts in medical–surgical nursing to undergraduate nursing students over the period of three college quarters. Levine also wished to move away from nursing education practices that were strongly procedurally oriented and refocus on active problem solving and individualized patient care (George, 2002).

The core, or central concept, of Levine's theory is *conservation* (Levine, 1989). When a person is in a state of conservation, it means that individual adaptive responses confront change productively, and with the least expenditure of effort, while preserving optimal function and identity. Conservation is achieved through successful activation of adaptive pathways and behaviors that are appropriate for the wide range of responses required by functioning human beings.

The specific adaptive responses that make conservation possible occur on many levels: molecular, physiologic, emotional, psychological, and social. These responses are based on three factors (Levine, 1989):

1. *Historicity* refers to the notion that adaptive responses are partially based on personal and genetic past history. Each individual is made up of a combination of personal and genetic history, and adaptive responses are the result of both. In other words, when assessing and supporting adaptive responses in clients, it is necessary for the nurse to take into account both personal and genetic factors when planning care.

2. *Specificity* refers to the fact that each system that makes up a human being has unique stimulus-response pathways. Responses are stimulated by specific stressors and are task oriented. Responses that are stimulated in multiple pathways tend to be synchronized and occur in a cascade of complementary (or detrimental, in some cases) reactions. For example, touching a hot stove will elicit a pain response, an inflammatory response at the site of injury, and an emotional response from the victim, all occurring at about the same time. The pain will cause the victim to rapidly withdraw the hand, resulting in the adaptive response of preventing further tissue damage. The inflammatory response at the site of injury will ultimately assist the body to repair and replace damaged tissue. The emotional response will aid the person in remembering what it is like to touch a hot stove so that the mistake will not be repeated in the future.

3. *Redundancy* describes the notion that if one system, or pathway, is unable to ensure adaptation, then another pathway may be able to take over and complete the job. This may be helpful when the response is corrective (e.g., the use of allergy shots over a lengthy period of time to diminish the effects of severe allergies by gradually desensitizing the immune system). However, redundancy may be detrimental, such as when previously failed responses are reestablished (e.g., when autoimmune conditions cause a person's own immune system to attack previously healthy tissue in the body).

The product of adaptation is conservation (George, 2002). The nurse's role in conservation is to support patient adaptation and to ensure that the least amount of patient effort is expended to achieve this state. Levine (1989) proposes four principles of conservation, each with unique pathways that are influenced by historicity, specificity, and redundancy, that nurses should practice:

1. *The conservation of energy of the individual.* Encourage rest so that the patient has the energy needed for baseline and healing functions.
2. *The conservation of the structural integrity of the individual.* Promote healing with as little further damage, or scarring, to the patient as possible.
3. *The conservation of personal integrity (retaining sense of self) of the individual.*
4. *The conservation of social integrity of the individual.* Preservation of old and, when needed, creation of new connections between patient and social entities outside of self.

Other assertions, or components, that appear in Levine's work include the following (George, 2002):

- Health and disease are patterns of adaptive change.
- The purpose of nursing is to take care of others when support of adaptive change is needed.
- Optimal health is the goal of conservation.
- The most successful adaptations are those that best support a state of conservation with the least amount of energy expended.
- A person who provides nursing care bears a heavy debt of responsibility when entering into another person's life during vulnerable times when illness has caused temporary dependency.

To summarize, Levine expressed the view that within the nurse–patient relationship a patient's state of health depends on the nurse-supported processes of adaptation. Effective adaptation leads to conservation, wherein the patient achieves his or her own unique optimal state of health with minimum energy expenditure. The goal of nursing care is to recognize, assist, promote, and support adaptive processes that benefit the patient.

A mandala design representing Levine's Conservation Model might include these components: the central, or focal, point is the concept of conservation. Immediately surrounding this central point are uniform shapes that represent the four principles of conservation. Around each of the four shapes are three identical circles that represent historicity, specificity, and redundancy. Evenly spaced beyond these central concepts are shapes representing supporting concepts that add clarity of meaning to the whole.

Theory in Action

Nursing theories are meant to stimulate and support knowledge development related to effectively exploring, predicting, describing, defining, and (sometimes) controlling nursing phenomena. Levine's work described a process that illuminated a balanced approach for aiding the progression of healing in medical–surgical patients. Her Conservation Model describes the interdependence of wholistic nursing care and patients' innate ability to achieve enhanced levels of wellness when nurses consciously support or assist adaptive responses. The two historical publications listed below, which are electronically accessible in the major databases, demonstrate Levine's theory in action:

Schaefer, K. M., & Shober, M. J. (1993). Fatigue associated with congestive heart failure: Use of Levine's Conservation Model. *Journal of Advance Nursing*, 18, 260–268. doi:10.1046/j.1365-2648.1993.18020260

   This article presents a study that utilized a descriptive approach, based on Levine's Conservation Model, to explore fatigue associated with heart failure. This study produced qualitative and quantitative data. The qualitative data explored sense of identity and self-worth. The quantitative data measured degree and understanding of fatigue and ability to engage in social activities. Findings were viewed in light of Levine's concept of adaptation. Implications for nursing focus on supporting a wholistic approach to patient care.

Mefford, L. C., & Alligood, M. R. (2011). Evaluating nurse staffing patterns and neonatal intensive care unit outcomes using Levine's Conservation Model of nursing. *Journal of Nursing Management*, 19, 998–1011. doi:10.1111/j.1365-2834.2011.01319

   In this study, the authors utilize Levine's Conservation Model as a framework to support the exploration of health and socioeconomic outcomes related to intensity and consistency of nursing care in a neonatal intensive care unit. Results indicated that maintaining consistency of nursing caregivers in relation to individual patients decreased duration of mechanical ventilation, length of stay, parenteral nutrition, and supplemental oxygen therapy.

Learning Activities

Locate and read the two articles listed above to see how nurses have used Levine's work.

1. To support deeper understanding of Levine's theory, envision and then create a mandala design on a blank sheet. Use the 10 questions listed in Chapter 10 as a guide. After completing the mandala, share your creation with your classmates.
2. Find websites or journal articles about Levine's theory. Words to use when performing a search might include:
   - Myra Estrin Levine
   - Conservation Model
   - Nursing theory

References

George, J. B. (2002). *Nursing theories: The base for professional nursing practice.* Upper Saddle River, NJ: Prentice Hall.

Levine, M. E. (1989). The conservation principles of nursing: Twenty years later. In J. P. Riehl-Sisca (Ed.), *Conceptual models for nursing practice* (3rd ed., pp. 325–337). Norwalk, CT: Appleton and Lange.

Betty Neuman's Systems Model

B etty Neuman was born in Ohio in 1924. She was a middle child with two brothers. When Betty was 11, her father died of kidney disease after several hospitalizations. Betty's father spoke highly of the nurses who cared for him in the hospital. Betty's mother was a rural midwife. Both of these factors played a part in inspiring Neuman to become a bedside nurse.

Neuman could not afford to attend nursing school directly after graduation from high school, so she worked as an aircraft instrument repair technician, draftsperson, and short-order cook while saving for her nursing education and helping to support her mother and younger brother. The creation of the Cadet Nurse Corps Program finally made it possible for Neuman to enter a hospital nursing school. She graduated with a diploma degree from People's Hospital in Akron, Ohio, in 1947. Neuman earned a Bachelor of Science degree in public health nursing in 1957 and a Master of Science degree in public health nursing and mental health nursing from the University of California, Los Angeles, in 1966. In 1985, Neuman was granted a doctorate degree in clinical psychology at Pacific Western University. Neuman also received an honorary doctorate from Grand Valley State in Michigan. Throughout her career as a nurse, Neuman worked in hospital and community health settings in a variety of staff and administrative positions. She also served as nursing faculty, chairing the nursing program from which she graduated.

The Neuman Systems Model was initially developed in the 1970s for use in nursing education. Neuman sought to create "a unifying focus for a wide range of nursing concerns . . . in particular, the model takes into account all variables affecting a client's possible or actual response to stressors and explains how system stability is achieved in relation to environmental stressors imposed on the client" (Neuman & Fawcett, 2002, p. 3).

Neuman's model was influenced by the General Systems Theory, which asserts that the world is made up of connected systems that exert influence on one another. If one system experiences disruption, it will affect all the other associated systems. Larger systems may be made up of layers of smaller systems. Envision a dipped chocolate candy with an inner core of vanilla fluff, then a layer of caramel over the fluff, followed by a layer of nuts over the caramel, then a layer of chocolate over the nuts, and ending with a layer of coconut over the chocolate. In Neuman's theory, the vanilla fluff would represent the core human being, with the outer layers representing levels of protection for the core.

Neuman's model was also influenced by the General Adaptation Syndrome (Hans Selye, 1907–1982). This syndrome asserts that humans and animals have a nonspecific response to stress that occurs in four stages (General Adaptation Syndrome, 1998):

1. *Alarm* occurs when there is an injury or prolonged stress to body or mind.
2. *Resistance* or *adaptation* occurs when various defense mechanisms of the mind and body are mobilized to address the stress.
3. *Exhaustion* results when the mind or body disintegrates.
4. *Adjustment* and *healing* occur when the mind or body effectively adapts to the stressor.

The General Adaptation Syndrome principles coupled with General Systems Model principles form the basis for the Neuman Systems Model approach of recognizing a structure "that depicts the parts and subparts and their interrelationship for the whole of a client as a complete system" (Neuman & Fawcett, 2002, p. 11). The concepts of *wholism* and *wellness* are discussed in relation to the theory in this way:

The philosophic base of the Neuman Systems Model encompasses wholism, a wellness orientation, client perception and motivation, and a dynamic systems perspective of energy and variable interaction with the environment to mitigate possible harm from internal and external stressors, while caregivers and clients form a partnership relationship to negotiate desired outcome goals for optimal health retention, restoration, and maintenance. (Neuman & Fawcett, 2002, p. 12)

Neuman's model recognizes the definitions of the following four concepts that are commonly used in nursing practice: client, environment, health, and nursing (Neuman & Fawcett, 2002):

- The person, family, group, or community is viewed as a *client* or *client system*. When discussing systems that contain more than one person, boundaries must be clearly defined with regard to who is included in the system and what relationships exist between system members. The client system is a composite of five interacting variables that are in various degrees of development. These variables are physiologic, psychological, sociocultural, developmental, and spiritual components.
- The *environment* includes all internal and external factors or influences that surround the client or client system.
- The concept of *health* is viewed as a continuum with wellness on one end and illness on the other. Health for the client or client system is equated with optimal system stability, or the best possible state of wellness at any given time.
- The major concern for *nursing* is to keep the client system stable through accurately assessing the effects and possible effects of stressors and assisting with client adjustments to obtain the highest degree of wellness possible at the time.

The following 10 statements summarize the overall approach of the Neuman Systems Model (Neuman & Fawcett, 2002):

1. Each individual client is a unique composite of innate responses that occur within a common range of "normal" as seen within most human beings.
2. The client is in dynamic, constant energy exchange with the environment.
3. Many known, unknown, and universal environmental stressors exist. Each differs in its potential for disturbing a client's usual stability level. Five interrelated variables that make up the client system may

affect the degree to which a client is protected from stressors. These five interrelated variables include physiologic, psychological, sociocultural, developmental, and spiritual aspects of the client system.

4. Each individual has evolved a normal range of responses to the environment that is referred to as the normal line of defense, or usual wellness/stability state. This normal line of defense evolves over time through coping with diverse stressors. The normal line of defense can be used as a standard from which to measure health deviation.

5. A flexible line of defense surrounds and protects the normal line of defense from invasion by stressors. An example of a component that would be a part of this defense would be consistent daily sleep patterns supporting rest, healing, and wellness. This flexible line of defense would be threatened by a change in sleep patterns, such as when a client becomes exhausted due to a lack of regular sleep while working rotating shifts and attending nursing school.

6. The client, whether ill or well, is a dynamic composite of the interrelationships of physiologic, psychological, sociocultural, developmental, and spiritual variables. Wellness is determined by the adequacy of energy available to support system stability.

7. Inside each client system, internal resistance factors function to stabilize and return the client to the usual, or possibly an improved, state of wellness following response to a stressor.

8. The nurse may be involved in the process of primary prevention, wherein general knowledge is applied in client assessment and preventive healthcare measures aimed at reducing the chance of possible stressors and resultant illness. Health-promotion activities fall within this category.

9. The nurse may be involved in secondary prevention activities, wherein there are symptoms of stress or illness apparent and treatment is provided to decrease the effects of the stressor.

10. The nurse may be involved in tertiary prevention activities, wherein adjustment following illness is supported, and maintenance activities aimed at returning the client system to stability move the client in a circular manner back to primary prevention.

Neuman expressed the view that it is helpful for nurses to approach nursing care using a structured, systems-oriented approach. By doing so, it is possible to discern interrelationships between multiple factors that dynamically influence health and wellness. Stressors cause system instability, and many variables affect a client's ability to regain health and stability after going through a period of stress. Using Neuman's approach, nurses have the opportunity to assess and appropriately address client stressors systematically and thoroughly so that optimal client wellness may be achieved in a variety of situations.

A mandala design representing the Neuman Systems Model might include these components: the central, or focal, point is the concept of a client or client system. The central point is large in the overall scheme of the design. Within the central point are shapes that represent the five interacting variables: physiologic, psychological, sociocultural, developmental, and spiritual components.

Arranged in concentric circles around the large central point are uniform shapes that represent the four definitions of *client, environment, health,* and *nursing.* Evenly spaced beyond these central concepts are shapes representing the supporting concepts that add clarity of meaning to the whole.

Theory in Action

Nursing theories are meant to stimulate and support knowledge development related to effectively exploring, predicting, describing, defining, and (sometimes) controlling nursing phenomena. Neuman's work proposed a structured approach to nursing care that sought to clarify how interrelated factors continually influence health and wellness. Carefully assessing these factors in light of system stability/instability and providing care focused on addressing stressors that cause instability support healing and wellness. The two publications listed below, one current and one historical, are electronically accessible in the major databases and demonstrate Neuman's theory in action:

Angosta, A. D., Ceria-Ulep, C. D., & Tse, A. M. (2014). Care delivery for Filipino Americans using the Neuman Systems Model. *Nursing Science Quarterly, 27,* 142–148. doi:10.1177/0894318414522605

In this article, Neuman's model provided a framework for exploring culturally appropriate preventive care for Filipino Americans at risk for cardiovascular disease.

Knight, J. B. (1990). The Betty Neuman Systems Model applied to practice: A client with multiple sclerosis. *Journal of Advanced Nursing*, 15(4), 447–455. doi:10.1111/j.1365-2648.1990.tb01838.x

This article demonstrates how Neuman's Systems Model applies to the care of clients with multiple sclerosis. An assessment tool based on Neuman's work is used to gather data related to a client who received a new diagnosis of multiple sclerosis. A Systems Model nursing care plan for this specific patient is created, implemented, and evaluated. Neuman's systems approach is validated in terms of supporting effective nursing process in this case.

Learning Activities

Locate and read the two articles listed above to see how nurses have used Neuman's work.

1. To support deeper understanding of Neuman's theory, envision and then create a mandala design on a blank sheet. Use the 10 questions listed in Chapter 10 as a guide. After completing the mandala, share your creation with your classmates.
2. Find websites or journal articles about Neuman's theory. Words to use when performing a search might include:
   • Betty Neuman
   • General Systems Theory
   • General Adaptation Syndrome
   • Neuman Systems Model

References

General Adaptation Syndrome. (1998). In *Mosby's Medical, Nursing, and Allied Health Dictionary* (5th ed.). St. Louis, MO: Mosby.

Neuman, B., & Fawcett, J. (2002). *The Neuman Systems Model* (4th ed.). Upper Saddle River, NJ: Prentice Hall.

Sister Callista Roy's Adaptation Model

Sister Callista Roy is a member of the Sisters of Saint Joseph of Carondelet. She was born in Los Angeles, California, on October 14, 1939, to loving parents. Her mother was a licensed vocational nurse, and Sr. Roy was the second oldest of 14 children, with 6 sisters and 7 brothers. She describes her children as "wonderful" and that she never felt "put upon" for having to share with so many but was rather proud to do so. Her love for nursing started when her brothers had whooping cough and she was left to care for them while her mother worked. She remembered the great sense of pride she felt at having done a good job. Learning to share and her faith in God influenced her life. She stated that she saw a lot of adaptation while she was growing up in such a large family and had many life examples before entering nursing school (Eichelberger, 2015).

In 1963, Roy earned a Bachelor of Arts degree in nursing from Mount Saint Mary's College in Los Angeles and a Master of Science in nursing in 1966 from the University of California, Los Angeles. Roy was awarded a Master of Arts degree in sociology in 1973 and a doctorate degree in sociology in 1977, both from the University of California. In the 1980s, Roy served on the faculties of several different institutions. She currently holds the position of professor and nurse theorist at Boston College, Boston, Massachusetts (Boston College, 2015).

While completing her MA degree, Roy was challenged by one of her nursing teachers, Dorothy E. Johnson, to create a conceptual model for nursing, and that is when she began to develop her Adaptation Model. The Roy Adaptation Model was first published in *Nursing Outlook* in 1970. Since that first journal article, Roy has published numerous books, chapters, and articles about the Roy Adaptation Model (Alligood & Tomey, 2010). Enthusiastic application and development of this model continue today.

Dr. Lisa Eichelberger interviewed Sr. Roy on May 1, 2015. During that meeting, Dr. Roy described the advice she would give new nurse theorists and how she got started in her early twenties describing the goal of nursing. She was able to formulate her adaptation theory by asking how a nurse helps patients live happy and healthy lives and how health and one's happiness are interrelated. She related that the basics of her theory have stayed the same over the past 50 years. Although the theory has been tested, refined, and expanded, the original elements have remained unchanged (Eichelberger, 2015).

The Roy Adaptation Model applies the concepts of *systems* and *adaptation* to nursing practice. In the context of Roy's work, the term *system* refers to a grouping of units that are related and connected, thus forming a unified whole. (A system may be an individual, family, group, community, or society.) *Adaptation* refers to effective coping mechanisms that promote integrity for a person, or group of persons, in terms of survival, growth, reproduction, and mastery. In general, Roy asserts that a person is a biophysical being (or system) in constant interaction with a changing environment and that a person has four different modes of adaptation. As internal and external environmental changes occur, needs change that may result in the necessity for active coping to restore integrity. Each client system (either person or group) has a zone that surrounds a variable level of adaptation. Stimuli that fall within the zone of adaptation result in positive adaptations that support integrity. Stimuli that fall outside the zone result in negative responses that do not support adaptation or integrity (Alligood & Tomey, 2010).

The four modes of adaptation that support integrity are as follows (Roy, 1984):

1. *Physiologic–physical* adaptation for an *individual* occurs when the five needs of oxygen, nutrition, elimination, activity/rest, and protection are met, in addition to adequate neurologic and endocrine function and

balanced fluids, electrolytes, and acid–base chemistry. Adaptation for a *group* includes adequate number of participants to achieve goals, shared productive capacities, adequate physical facilities, and fiscal resources.

2. *Self-concept group identity* adaptation for an *individual* occurs when psychic and spiritual integrity promotes a sense of purpose, unity, and meaning in the universe. Adaptation for a *group* includes group identity maintained through honestly shared relations, goals, and values, coupled with a shared sense of achievement.

3. *Role function* adaptation for an *individual* includes knowing who one is in relation to others and involves the use of various adaptive modes suited to the unique multiple roles expected of each individual. Adaptation for a *group* involves enactment of varied role responsibilities that ultimately support the achievement of common goals.

4. *Interdependence* adaptation for an *individual* includes the giving and receiving of love, participating in satisfying relationships, and engaging in meaningful communication. Adaptation for a *group* includes involvement in continually maturing collective relationships and achieving adequate food, shelter, health, and security through interdependence with other group members.

Four major concepts constitute the Roy Adaptation Model:

1. *Humans are wholistic, adaptive systems as both individuals and groups.* "As living systems, persons are in constant interaction with their environments. Between the system and the environment occurs an exchange of information, matter, and energy. Characteristics of a system include inputs, outputs, controls, and feedback" (George, 2002, p. 298).

2. The *environment* is made up of internal and external stimuli from around the individual or group system. Environment includes "all conditions, circumstances, and influences that surround and affect the development and behavior of humans as adaptive systems, with particular consideration of person and earth resources" (Roy & Andrews, 1999, p. 52).

3. *Health* is defined as "a state and process of being and becoming an integrated whole as a human being. . . . [*Integrity* is defined as] soundness or unimpaired condition leading to wholeness" (Roy & Andrews, 1999, p. 54).

4. The *goal of nursing* is the promotion of the four modes of adaptation, thereby supporting the overall integrity of the human adaptive system. Nurses also seek to reduce ineffective responses through anticipating and addressing potential concerns and also effectively attending to current concerns (George, 2002; Roy & Andrews, 1999).

Roy's Adaptation Model is particularly suited for use with the traditional nursing process. Following is a version of the nursing process as it might be viewed within the context of the Roy Adaptation Model (George, 2002):

- *Assessment of client(s) behavior* involves observing for "actions or reactions under specified circumstances. It can be observable or nonobservable" (Roy & Andrews, 1999, p. 67). This activity is consistent with the notion of gathering output from a human system.
- *Assessment of stimuli* involves analyzing patterns of client output to identify ineffective adaptive responses that require nursing intervention.
- *Nursing diagnosis* is created by the nurse and represents an interpretation of how well the human system is adapting to whatever condition or situation brought them to the point of assessment.
- *Goal setting* involves clearly stating the desired outcomes of nursing care, including desired client behavior, specific nature of any expected changes, and the time frame in which this will occur.
- *Interventions* "are planned with the purpose of altering stimuli or strengthening adaptive processes. The nurse plans specific activities to alter the selected stimuli appropriately" (George, 2002, p. 320).
- *Evaluation* assesses the effectiveness of the interventions and involves active input from both the nurse and the client. Specifically, "goal behaviors are compared to the client's output responses, and movement toward or away from goal achievement is determined. If the goals have not been met, then the nursing process begins again" (George, 2002, p. 321).

Roy's work has a broad scientific and philosophical foundation that provides the underpinnings of this model. Philosophically, Roy's model supports a "focus on awareness and the notion of eliminating false consciousness, enlightenment to reach self-control, balance, and quietude, and the reclamation of earthly creation as the core of faith" (Roy & Andrews, 1999, p. 35). The following are an additional 10 scientific and philosophical assumptions that influence Roy's Adaptation Model (George, 2002; Roy & Andrews, 1999):

1. Systems of matter and energy progress to higher levels of self-organization.
2. Consciousness and meaning demonstrate person–environment integration.
3. Awareness of self and environment is rooted in thinking and feeling, and thinking and feeling mediate human actions.
4. System relationships include acceptance, protection, and fostering of interdependence.
5. Persons and the earth have common patterns and integral relationships.
6. Human consciousness has the power to transform persons and environment.
7. Persons have mutual relationships with the world and God.
8. Human meaning is rooted in an omega-point convergence of the universe.
9. God is revealed in creation.
10. Persons are accountable for the process of transforming the universe.

In summary, the Roy Adaptation Model proposes a structure for nursing practice that focuses on the human being as an adaptive system. This human adaptive system continually interacts with stimuli. On the occasions that a human being, or group of human beings, is unable to maintain wholeness or integrity with respect to necessary life processes, nursing intervention can help to restore adaptation, effective coping, and ultimately optimal health. Nurses work primarily in the realm of supporting adaptive responses, whereas the medical profession focuses more on the health–illness continuum. With conscious collaboration, the two disciplines are able to provide effective client support in times of medical need.

A mandala design representing the Roy Adaptation Model might include these components: the central, or focal, point is the concept of *client/client system*. The central point is large in the overall scheme of the design. Within the central point are shapes that represent the four modes of adaptation: *physiologic/physical, self-concept/group identity, role function*, and *interdependence*. Around the large central point, uniform shapes are intertwined that represent the four major concepts of the model: *client* as adaptive system, *environment* as stimulus, *health* as adaptation/wholistic integrity, and *nursing* as a support to adaptation. In a large circle surrounding these central concepts are shapes that represent each of the steps in the nursing process. Surrounding and enveloping the entire design are shapes representing the supporting scientific and philosophical concepts.

Theory in Action

Nursing theories are meant to stimulate and support knowledge development related to effectively exploring, predicting, describing, defining, and (sometimes) controlling nursing phenomena. Roy's Adaptation Model offers a structure for considering the nurse's role in supporting the adaptive responses of patients. She advocated collaboration and interdisciplinary work during a time when this concept was not at the forefront; however, her work foreshadowed what has become a central theme in health care today. The two publications listed below, which are electronically accessible in the major databases, demonstrate Roy's theory in action:

Cypress, B. S. (2011). Patient-family-nurse intensive care unit experience: A Roy Adaptation Model–based qualitative study. *Qualitative Research Journal*, 11(2), 3–16. doi:10.3316/QRJ1102003

In this article, the author describes a phenomenological study that explored the experiences of patients, families, and nurses in an intensive care unit during critical illness. Analysis of the data produced themes that reflected concepts from the Roy Adaptation Model and highlighted a shared experience of interdependence that resulted in personal growth, empowerment, and transformation.

Barone, S. H., & Waters, K. (2012). Coping and adaptation in adults living with spinal cord injury. *Journal of Neuroscience Nursing*, 44(5), 271–283. doi:10.1097/JNN.0b01 3e3182666203

In this article, the authors discuss a descriptive study that assessed coping as it related to biopsychosocial adaptation in patients with spinal cord injuries. Multiple variables related to age, level of injury, perceived control, and hardiness influenced biopsychosocial adaptation.

Learning Activities

Locate and read the two articles listed above to see how nurses have used Roy's work.

1. To support deeper understanding of Roy's theory, envision and then create a mandala design on a blank sheet. Use the 10 questions listed in Chapter 10 as a guide. After completing the mandala, share your creation with your classmates.
2. Find websites or journal articles about Roy's theory. Words to use when performing a search might include:
   • Sister Callista Roy
   • Systems theory
   • Nursing process
   • Adaptation Model

References

Alligood, M. R., & Tomey, A. M. (2010). *Nursing theorists and their work* (7th ed.). Maryland Heights, MO: Mosby.

Boston College William F. Connell School of Nursing. (2015). Sr. Callista Roy, PhD, RN, FAAN. Retrieved from https://www.bc.edu/schools/son/faculty/featured/theorist .html

Eichelberger, L. (2015, May 1). Dr. Eichelberger's interview with Sr. Callista Roy. [Video]. Retrieved from https://www.youtube.com/watch?v=WJTtld5McsI &feature=youtu.b

George, J. B. (2002). *Nursing theories: The base for professional nursing practice.* Upper Saddle River, NJ: Prentice Hall.

Roy, C. (1984). *Introduction to nursing: An adaptation model* (2nd ed.). Upper Saddle River, NJ: Prentice Hall.

Roy, C., & Andrews, H. A. (1999). *The Roy Adaptation Model* (2nd ed.). Stamford, CT: Appleton & Lange.

Dorothea Orem's Self-Care Model

Dorothea Orem was born in Baltimore, Maryland, in 1914. Orem earned her diploma in nursing in the 1930s. In 1939, she earned her Bachelor of Science degree in nursing education, which was followed by a Master of Science degree in nursing education in 1945 from the Catholic University of America. She has received many professional awards and honorary degrees. Over her long professional career, Orem has worked as a staff nurse, a private duty nurse, a nursing faculty member, an administrator, and a consultant. Orem's nursing concept of self-care was first published in 1959. She continued to develop this theory and in 1980 published the first edition of *Nursing: Concepts of Practice*, the sixth edition appearing in 2001. Orem worked as a nurse consultant in Savannah, Georgia, until her death on June 22, 2007, at the age of 92.

Orem's Self-Care Model is generally stated as follows (Orem, 2001, p. 82):

The condition that validates the existence of a requirement for nursing in an adult is the health-associated absence of the ability to maintain continuously that amount and quality of self-care that is therapeutic in sustaining life and health, in recovering from disease or injury, or in coping with their effects. With children, the condition is the inability of the parent (or guardian) associated with the child's health state to maintain continuously for the child the amount and quality of care that is therapeutic.

Orem's Self-Care Model is composed of the three interrelated concepts of self-care, self-care deficit, and nursing systems (George, 2002).

Self-care involves the four aspects of self-care, self-care agency, basic conditioning factors, and therapeutic self-care demand. *Self-care* is what people plan and do on their own behalf to maintain life, health, and well-being. When self-care is effectively performed, it helps maintain structural integrity and human functioning and contributes to human development (George, 2002; Orem, 2001). *Self-care agency* is a person's acquired ability to engage in self-care. Self-care agency is affected by *basic conditioning factors* that include age, gender, developmental and health states, sociocultural factors, healthcare system factors, family system factors, patterns of living, environmental factors, and adequacy and availability of resources. *Therapeutic self-care demand* refers to what is needed at various times in a person's life when health care is required to meet self-care needs through the use of appropriate actions and interventions (George, 2002). Orem identified the following primary needs that must be met by human beings to ensure adequate self-care (George, 2002; Orem, 2001):

1. Sufficient intake of air, water, and food
2. Adequate care and functioning of elimination
3. Balance between activity and rest
4. Balance between solitude and social interaction
5. Prevention of hazards to human life, functioning, and well-being
6. Promotion of functioning and appropriate development within social groups in accord with human potential, limitations, and the human desire to be normal

When a person is in the position of needing medical care to diagnose or correct an illness, adequate self-care also includes the following (Orem, 2001):

1. Seeking and securing medical help when needed
2. Responsibly attending to the effects and results of pathologic conditions
3. Effectively carrying out prescribed interventions
4. Responsibly attending to the regulation of effects resulting from prescribed interventions
5. Accepting the fact that sometimes self or others need medical help when faced with certain life challenges
6. Learning to live productively with the effects of pathologic conditions and treatments while promoting continued personal development

Self-care deficit results when adults or parents with dependent children are incapable of providing continuously effective self-care. Nursing care may be required if there is a need for education to enhance self-care abilities, if there is a current deficit in self-care abilities, or if it is anticipated that self-care abilities will decrease in the future. The five methods of helping, to be used alone or in combination when there is concern over a self-care deficit, are as follows (Orem, 2001):

1. Acting for or doing for another
2. Guiding and directing
3. Providing physical or psychological support
4. Providing and maintaining an environment that supports personal development
5. Teaching

Nursing systems are designed by nurses based on an assessment of the individual's self-care needs. "If there is a deficit between what the individual can do (self-care agency) and what needs to be done to maintain optimum functioning (therapeutic self-care demand), then nursing is required" (George, 2002, p. 131). Orem has described three kinds of nursing systems that are meant to meet the variable needs of individual situations. These three systems include (George, 2002):

1. The *wholly compensatory system* is one in which patient action is limited and the nurse accomplishes most of what is required to maintain therapeutic self-care, compensates for the patient's inability to engage in self-care, and supports and protects the patient.
2. The *partially compensatory system* is one in which the patient and nurse work together to meet self-care requirements, with the patient performing some of the tasks necessary for successful self-care and the nurse performing whatever else is required.
3. The *supportive-educative system* is one in which the patient provides necessary self-care, and the nurse and patient work together to regulate the exercise and development of self-care agency.

These three combined concepts of self-care, self-care deficit, and nursing systems make up a general Self-Care Model with a three-step nursing process that can be compared with the widely used *nursing process*. Orem's three steps follow, with corresponding nursing process steps provided in parentheses (George, 2002):

1. Diagnosis and prescription includes determining why nursing care is needed through careful analysis and interpretation of information gathered while assessing the patient. This is the step when nurses make professional judgments regarding what care to provide (assessment and nursing diagnosis, including desired outcomes).
2. Design of a nursing system and plan for delivery of care to achieve desired outcomes (plans with scientific rationale).
3. Production and management of nursing systems (implementation and evaluation).

In summary, Orem's Self-Care Model describes a structure wherein the nurse assists the client, where needed, to maintain an adequate level of self-care. The degree of nursing care and intervention depends on the degree to which the client is able (or unable) to meet self-care needs. This theory is structured in such a way that the concepts are straightforward to understand and apply. The simplicity of wording, coupled with an uncanny resonance with everyday nursing activities, has ensured its broad popularity and use in many areas of nursing.

A mandala design representing Orem's model might contain these components: there is a large central point divided into three lobes representing *self-care*, *self-care deficit*, and *nursing systems*. Streaming outward from the self-care lobe is a shape that encompasses the four concepts of self-care, self-care agency, basic conditioning factors, and therapeutic self-care demand. Streaming outward from the self-care deficit lobe is a shape that encompasses the five methods of helping. Streaming outward from the nursing systems lobe is a shape that encompasses the three systems of nursing care. Encircling the periphery of the design are Orem's three nursing process steps.

Theory in Action

Nursing theories are meant to stimulate and support knowledge development related to effectively exploring, predicting, describing, defining, and (sometimes) controlling nursing phenomena. Orem's work defined nursing in terms of identifying and managing multiple variables while helping patients toward independence and wellness. Two publications listed below, which are electronically accessible in the major databases, demonstrate Orem's theory in action:

Wilson, J., & Gramling, L. (2009). The application of Orem's Self-Care Model to burn care. *Journal of Burn Care and Research*, 30(5), 852–858. doi:10.1097/BCR.0b013e3181b48a2d

In this article, Wilson and Gramling applied Orem's Self-Care Model to the process of nurses caring for burn patients. They focused on correlating Orem's three systems (wholly compensatory, partially compensatory, and supportive/educative) with the unique care needs of burn patients and their families. The authors assert that deliberative use of Orem's Self-Care Model in burn nursing will facilitate professionalism and begin needed dialogue related to theory application in this specific specialty area.

Altay, N., & Cavusoglu, H. (2013). Using Orem's Self-Care Model for asthmatic adolescents. *Journal for Specialists in Pediatric Nursing*, 18, 233–242. doi:10.1111/jspn.12032

This article presents results of a study that was undertaken to determine the effect of utilizing Orem's Self-Care Model to guide home healthcare nursing interventions for adolescents with asthma. Results indicated that use of Orem's model supported favorable patient outcomes in the study group.

Learning Activities

Locate and read the two articles listed above to see how nurses have used Orem's work.

1. To support deeper understanding of Orem's theory, envision and then create a mandala design on a blank sheet. Use the 10 questions listed in Chapter 10 as a guide. After completing the mandala, share your creation with your classmates.

2. Find websites or journal articles about Orem's theory. Words to use when performing a search might include:
   - Dorothy Orem
   - Self-Care Model

References

George, J. B. (2002). *Nursing theories: The base for professional nursing practice*. Upper Saddle River, NJ: Prentice Hall.

Orem, D. E. (2001). *Nursing: Concepts and practice* (6th ed.). St. Louis, MO: Mosby.

Madeleine Leininger's Culture Care: Diversity and Universality Theory

Madeleine Leininger was born in Sutton, Nebraska. In 1948, she received her diploma in nursing from St. Anthony's School of Nursing in Denver, Colorado. In 1950, she earned a Bachelor of Science degree from St. Scholastica (Benedictine College) in Atchison, Kansas, and in 1954 earned a Master of Science degree in psychiatric and mental health nursing from the Catholic University of America in Washington, D.C. In 1965, she was awarded a doctorate in cultural and social anthropology from the University of Washington, Seattle (Tomey & Alligood, 2002).

Early in her career as a nurse, Leininger recognized the importance of the concept of "caring" in nursing. Frequent statements of appreciation from patients for care received prompted Leininger to focus on "care" as being a central component of nursing. During the 1950s, while working in a child guidance home, Leininger experienced what she describes as a cultural shock when she realized that recurrent behavioral patterns in children appeared to have a cultural basis. Leininger identified a lack of cultural and care knowledge as the missing link to nursing's understanding of the many variations required in patient care to support compliance, healing, and wellness (George, 2002). These insights were the beginnings (in the 1950s) of a new construct and phenomenon related to nursing care called *transcultural nursing*.

Leininger is the founder of the transcultural nursing movement in education research and practice. In 1995, Leininger defined transcultural nursing as

> . . .a substantive area of study and practice focused on comparative cultural care (caring) values, beliefs, and practices of individuals or groups of similar or different cultures with the goal of providing culture-specific and universal nursing care practices in promoting health or well-being or to help people to face unfavorable human conditions, illness, or death in culturally meaningful ways. (p. 58)

The practice of transcultural nursing addresses the cultural dynamics that influence the nurse–client relationship. Because of its focus on this specific aspect of nursing, a theory was needed to study and explain outcomes of this type of care. Leininger creatively developed the Theory of Culture Care: Diversity and Universality with the goal to provide culturally congruent wholistic care.

Some scholars might place this theory in the middle-range classification. Leininger holds that it is not a grand theory because it has particular dimensions to assess for a total picture. It is a wholistic and comprehensive approach, which has led to broader nursing practice applications than is traditionally expected with a middle-range, reductionist approach (Penny Glynn, personal communication, September 12, 2003).

Leininger's theory is to provide care measures that are in harmony with an individual's or group's cultural beliefs, practices, and values. In the 1960s, she coined the term *culturally congruent care*, which is the primary goal of transcultural nursing practice. Culturally congruent care is possible when the following occurs within the nurse–client relationship:

> Together the nurse and the client creatively design a new or different care lifestyle for the health or well-being of the client. This mode requires the use of both generic and professional knowledge and ways to fit such diverse ideas into nursing care actions and goals. Care knowledge and skill are often repatterned for the best interest of the clients. . . . Thus all care modalities require *coparticipation of the nurse and clients (consumers) working together* to identify, plan, implement, and evaluate each caring mode for culturally congruent nursing care. These modes can stimulate nurses to design nursing actions and decisions using new knowledge and culturally based ways to provide meaningful and satisfying wholistic care to individuals, groups or institutions. (Leininger, 1991, p. 44)

Leininger developed new terms for the basic tenets of her theory. These definitions and the tenets are important to understand. Understanding such key terms is crucial to understanding the theory. Below is a basic summary of the tenets that are essential to understand Leininger's theory (summarized from Leininger, 2001, pp. 46–47):

- *Care* is to assist others with real or anticipated needs in an effort to improve a human condition of concern or to face death.
- *Caring* is an action or activity directed toward providing *care*.
- *Culture* refers to learned, shared, and transmitted values, beliefs, norms, and lifeways of a specific individual or group that guide their thinking, decisions, actions, and patterned ways of living.
- *Cultural care* refers to multiple aspects of *culture* that influence and enable a person or group to improve their human condition or to deal with illness or death.
- *Cultural care diversity* refers to the differences in meanings, values, or acceptable modes of care within or between different groups of people.
- *Cultural care universality* refers to common *care* or similar meanings that are evident among many cultures.
- *Nursing* is a learned profession with a disciplined focused on care phenomena.
- *Worldview* refers to the way people tend to look at the world or universe in creating a personal view of what life is about.
- *Cultural and social structure dimensions* include factors related to religion, social structure, political/legal concerns, economics, educational patterns, and the use of technologies, cultural values, and ethnohistory that influence cultural responses of human beings within a cultural context.
- *Health* refers to a state of well-being that is culturally defined and valued by a designated culture.
- *Cultural care preservation or maintenance* refers to nursing care activities that help people of particular cultures to retain and use core cultural care values related to healthcare concerns or conditions.
- *Cultural care accommodation or negotiation* refers to creative nursing actions that help people of a particular culture adapt to or negotiate with others in the healthcare community in an effort to attain the shared goal of an optimal health outcome for client(s) of a designated culture.
- *Cultural care repatterning or restructuring* refers to therapeutic actions taken by culturally competent nurse(s) or family. These actions enable or

assist a client to modify personal health behaviors toward beneficial outcomes while respecting the client's cultural values.

Several specific assumptions inherent in this theory support the theory premises and Leininger's use of the terms described above. These assumptions are the philosophical basis of Culture Care: Diversity and Universality theory. They add meaning, depth, and clarity to the overall focus to arrive at culturally competent nursing care. The following are distilled from Leininger's work and preceded use by other nurses, who in recent years have begun to value and employee these ideas and the theory. These statements are derived from Leininger's key sources (Leininger 1978, 1981, 1991, 1995, 2002, and most specifically, 2001, pp. 44–45):

- Care is the essence and central focus of nursing.
- Caring is essential for health and well-being, healing, growth, survival, and also for facing illness or death.
- Culture care is a broad, wholistic perspective to guide nursing care practices.
- Nursing's central purpose is to serve human beings in health, illness, and dying.
- There can be no curing without the giving and receiving of care.
- Culture care concepts have both different and similar aspects among all cultures of the world.
- Every human culture has folk remedies, professional knowledge, and professional care practices that vary. The nurse must identify and address these factors consciously with each client in order to provide wholistic and culturally congruent care.
- Cultural care values, beliefs, and practices are influenced by worldview and language, as well as religious, spiritual, social, political, educational, economic, technological, ethnohistorical, and environmental factors.
- Beneficial, healthy, satisfying culturally based nursing care enhances the well-being of clients.
- Culturally beneficial nursing care can occur only when cultural care values, expressions, or patterns are known and used appropriately and knowingly by the nurse providing care.
- Clients who experience nursing care that fails to be reasonably congruent with the client's cultural beliefs and values will show signs of stress, cultural conflict, noncompliance, and ethical moral concerns.

In synthesizing the information contained in the defining terms and assumptions just presented, a broad definition emerges of a culturally competent nurse who

- Consciously addresses the fact that culture affects all nurse–client exchanges
- Asks, with compassion and clarity, each client what their cultural practices and preferences are
- Incorporates the client's personal, social, environmental, and cultural needs and beliefs into the plan of care whenever possible
- Respects and appreciates cultural diversity, and strives to increase knowledge and sensitivity associated with this essential nursing concern

In summary, nurses who understand and value the practice of culturally competent care are able to effect positive changes in healthcare practices for clients of designated cultures. Sharing a cultural identity requires a knowledge of transcultural nursing concepts and principles, along with an awareness of current research findings. Culturally competent nursing care can occur only when client beliefs and values are thoughtfully and skillfully incorporated into nursing care plans. Caring is the core of nursing. Culturally competent nursing guides the nurse to provide optimal wholistic, culturally based care. These practices also help the client to care for himself or herself and others within a familiar, supportive, and meaningful cultural context. Continual improvement and expansion of modern technologies and other nursing and general science knowledge are integrated into practice if they are appropriate. Today nurses are faced daily with unprecedented cultural diversity because of the increasing number of immigrants and refugees. Commitment to learning and practicing culturally competent care offers great satisfaction and many other rewards to those who can provide wholistic supportive care to all patients (Leininger 1991, 2002).

A mandala design representing Leininger's model might be viewed as a mandala of the primary colors arranged in overlapping circles. The places where the colors overlap create new colors; for example, the place where blue and red overlap creates the color purple. The primary colors represent cohesive cultures that intermingle with others in a limited way, thereby maintaining a strong group identity. The mixed colors represent different cultures that are influenced by multiple cultures. All of the interwoven colors represent many cultures interacting to varying degrees and forming functional communities in an ever-widening circle of interaction and inclusion. The shapes in the design would have symmetry and balance to suggest unity and harmony among them.

Theory in Action

Nursing theories are meant to stimulate and support knowledge development related to effectively exploring, predicting, describing, defining, and (sometimes) controlling nursing phenomena. Leininger's work was groundbreaking in that she created a theory that acknowledged the pivotal role that culture plays in health care. She asserted that nurses must tailor care to meet the cultural needs of the patient. At the time the theory was first being developed, this was a radical departure from the accepted approach that the patient should be expected to mold to the expectations and directives of healthcare providers. The two historical publications listed below, which are electronically accessible in the major databases, demonstrate Leininger's theory in action:

Rosenbaum, J. N. (1990). Cultural care of older Greek Canadian widows within Leininger's theory of culture care. *Journal of Transcultural Nursing*, 2(1), 37–47. doi:10.1177/104365969000200106

This article presents a study in which cultural care themes were identified within a group that comprised older Greek Canadian widows. Results described two cultural patterns: (1) cultural care within this group was demonstrated by reciprocation, concern, love, companionship, family protection, hospitality, and helping; and (2) continuity of cultural care diminished the spousal care void and supported wellness.

Luna, L. (1994). Care and cultural context of Lebanese Muslim immigrants: Using Leininger's theory. *Journal of Transcultural Nursing*, 5(2), 12–20. doi:10.1177/104365969400500203

This article is about a study aimed at analyzing the meanings and experiences of care in a group of Lebanese Muslims. Inquiry focused on informant experiences in hospital, clinic, and home settings, as influenced by worldview, social structure, and cultural context. Three care contexts reflected care as a religious obligation in Islam, care as equal but different gender role responsibilities, and care as individual and collective honor.

Learning Activities

Locate and read the two articles listed above to see how nurses have used Leininger's work.

1. To support deeper understanding of Leininger's theory, envision and then create a mandala design on a blank sheet. Use the 10 questions listed in Chapter 10 as a guide.
2. Share the mandala you created with classmates.
3. Find websites about Leininger's theory or search for journal articles. Words to use when performing a search might include:
   - Madeleine Leininger
   - Cultural care
   - Diversity
   - Transcultural Nursing Care

References

George, J. B. (2002). *Nursing theories: The base for professional nursing practice.* Upper Saddle River, NJ: Prentice Hall.

Leininger, M. (1978). *Transcultural nursing: Concepts, theories, and practices.* New York, NY: John Wiley.

Leininger, M. (1981). *Care: An essential human need.* Detroit, MI: Wayne State University Press.

Leininger, M. (1991). *Culture care diversity and universality: A theory of nursing.* New York, NY: National League for Nursing Press.

Leininger, M. (1995). *Transcultural nursing: Concepts, theories, and practices* (2nd ed.). Blacklic, OH: McGraw-Hill and Greyden Press.

Leininger, M. (2001). *Culture care diversity and universality: A theory of nursing.* Sudbury, MA: Jones and Bartlett Publishers.

Leininger, M. (2002). *Transcultural nursing: Concepts, theories, research, and practices* (3rd ed.). Blacklic, OH: McGraw-Hill Professional.

Tomey, A. M., & Alligood, M. R. (2002). *Nursing theorists and their work* (5th ed.). St. Louis, MO: Mosby.

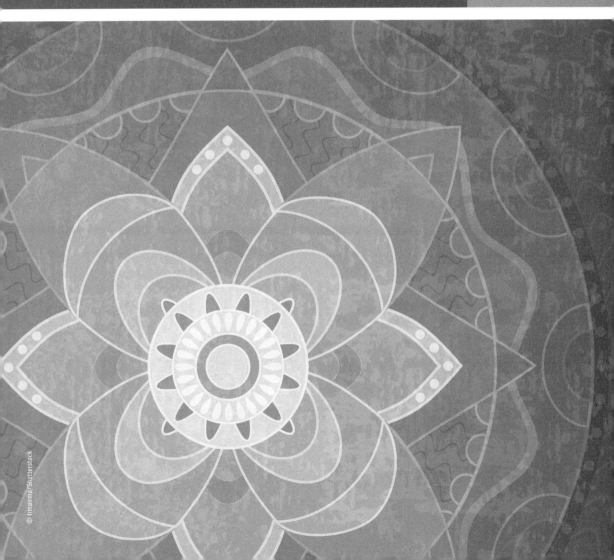

Theories About Specific Nursing Actions, Processes, or Concepts: Middle-Range Theories

PART

IV

Envisioning Theories Through Origami Art

Theories about specific nursing actions, processes, or concepts (*middle-range theories*) seek to define and provide direction for specific nursing activities. Middle-range theories are those in which nursing topics are most readily identifiable, and nurses who wish to follow the actions or steps described in a theory may do so. Nurses also may be able to replicate or simulate the experience described in the theory. For example, a middle-range theory might propose that there are six steps to productive mentoring relationships between experienced nurses and new nurses. It would be relatively straightforward for a nurse manager, using the theory as a guide, to institute and evaluate the effectiveness of using this six-step approach for mentoring new hires in her unit. If the approach turns out to be effective, then the nurse manager has implemented a valuable tool to enhance consistency of training for new hires. If the approach turns out to be less than helpful, then knowledge has been gained regarding applicability of the theory in this setting. Information has also been provided about mentoring techniques that may not be helpful within this nurse manager's particular pool of staff nurses. With either outcome, useful knowledge has been generated that will clarify for the staff nurses or the manager which approach might be most useful when mentoring new hires.

Envision origami when exploring theories that seek to describe a specific nursing action or process (middle-range theory). Origami is the art of following specific steps for folding paper into recognizable designs or forms (see **Color Plates 21** and **22** in the color insert). The word *origami* is Japanese; however, people in all cultures have engaged in paper folding since the invention of mass-produced paper roughly a century ago. In the United States, many children experiment with the process of folding paper into readily identifiable objects such as party hats, sailboats, and airplanes.

The art of origami consists of steps or actions that are meant to lead to a specific outcome or result, and, likewise, middle-range theories consist of steps or actions that are meant to lead to a specific outcome or result. In nursing, the steps lead to a readily identifiable outcome related to care, and in origami the steps lead to a readily identifiable concrete object. In either case, carefully planned steps and actions are meant to lead to a concrete, desired outcome.

To create origami, one begins with a flat, square piece of paper that does not resemble a recognizable object. With careful step-by-step folding, the paper becomes something recognizable, such as an animal, flower, insect, boat, or airplane. The idea is simple: decide what object will be evident after the folding is complete, such as an airplane, and then carefully fold the paper over and over again, until the airplane is done. If a friend folds a particularly good airplane, the best way to figure out how to make one just like it is to carefully unfold the creation and then follow the folds (or steps) to re-create it, learning how to replicate the design. Nursing research based on middle-range theories follows this same process of choosing a desired outcome and then following the steps provided in the theory to try to re-create the desired result.

Using a piece of copy paper or wrapping paper, create the origami airplane as shown in **Figure 16.1**.

The steps involved in the exploration of middle-range theories are similar to the steps involved in producing origami. The following are steps to use when exploring middle-range theories; the corresponding origami steps are in italics:

1. Identify what the concrete outcome of interest is, for example, effective mentoring. *Identify what object will be produced, for example, a sailboat.*
2. Determine what processes or steps, for example, those meant to lead to effective mentoring, are outlined in the theory. *Find a pattern or series of fold sequences for transforming a sheet of paper into a sailboat.*

Origami Art

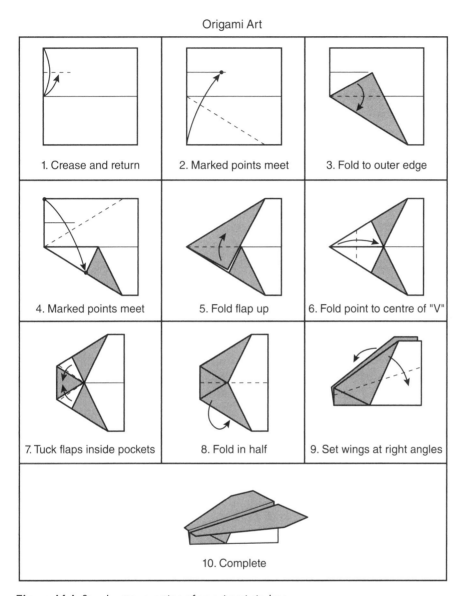

Figure 16.1 Step-by-step creation of an origami airplane.

3. Through reflection and personal experience, assess whether the process or series of steps outlined in the theory resonate with personal understanding of effective nurse mentoring. *After completing all of the folds in the origami pattern, assess how closely the creation resembles your understanding of what a sailboat should look like.*

4. If the steps or processes outlined in the theory do not appear to match personal/professional experiences with the phenomenon of nurse mentoring, then explore a different theory or create a new one. *If the completed creation does not look like a sailboat, try another pattern or create a new one.*

Try creating some traditional origami art. Be mindful of the importance of each fold (or step) in completing the finished object. **Figure 16.2** presents another traditional pattern to try.

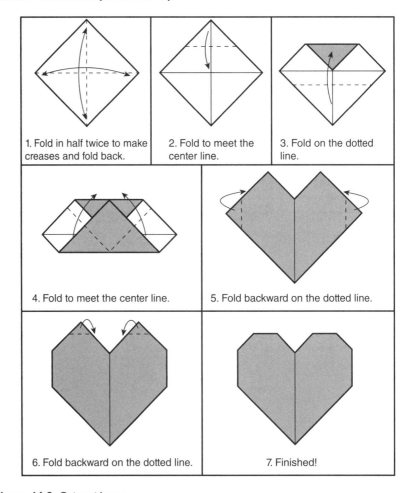

Figure 16.2 Origami heart.

When reading about theories that address a specific nursing action or process (a middle-range theory), ask yourself these questions:

1. What is the purpose of this theory? What is it meant to describe?
2. What are the steps outlined by the theory to achieve the desired result?
3. Are there a sufficient number of steps, and are they explained well enough that others would be able to replicate the desired result?
4. Does the overall pattern and resulting object, or process, resonate with personal/professional nursing experience?
5. What nursing environments would be appropriate to use this theory in?
6. Where would it *not be appropriate* to use the theory?
7. Would it be productive to share this theory with others who work in environments where it might fit?

Ida Jean Orlando-Pelletier's Nursing Process Theory

Ida Jean Orlando-Pelletier was born August 12, 1926, to Italian immigrants. She grew up during the Depression and received a diploma in nursing in 1947 from New York Medical College, Lower Fifth Avenue Hospital School of Nursing. She earned a Bachelor of Science degree in public health nursing in 1951 from St. John's University in Brooklyn, New York. In 1954, Orlando-Pelletier earned her Master of Arts degree in mental health consultation from Columbia University Teachers College. During her years of educational progression, Orlando-Pelletier worked in a variety of nursing settings. After completing her Master of Arts, Orlando-Pelletier taught for 8 years at the Yale School of Nursing in New Haven, Connecticut. While at Yale, Orlando-Pelletier was a research associate and principal investigator of a federal project grant entitled "Integration of Mental Health Concepts in a Basic Curriculum," during which time she collected data while observing students interact with patients and other members of the educational and healthcare team. After analyzing these data, Orlando-Pelletier reported her findings in a book published in 1961 entitled *The Dynamic Nurse–Patient Relationship: Function, Process, and Principles of Professional Nursing Practice* (Orlando, 1961/1990). Since its initial publication, the book has been published in five other languages in addition to English. The information in this book forms the foundation of Orlando-Pelletier's Nursing Process theory (Tomey & Alligood, 2002).

Orlando-Pelletier's Nursing Process theory is based on the premise that the nurse–patient relationship is reciprocal, meaning that the actions of one affect the other. Orlando-Pelletier is one of the first nursing leaders to recognize the pivotal importance of patient participation and intelligent nurse deliberation in the nursing process. Orlando-Pelletier also believes that the nursing profession is distinct from the medical profession and that "nursing action is derived from the patient's immediate experience and immediate needs for help" (Tomey & Alligood, 2002, p. 400). Said another way, Orlando-Pelletier's theory asserts that "nursing is unique and independent because it concerns itself with an individual's need for help, real or potential, in an immediate situation. The process by which nursing resolves this helplessness is interactive and is pursued in a disciplined manner that requires training. She [Orlando-Pelletier] believes one's actions should be based on rationale, not protocols" (George, 2002, p. 191). Orlando-Pelletier's work is considered to be a middle-range theory because it proposes a specific process of deliberative, intentional one-to-one interaction between the nurse and patient to support optimal nursing care directed at addressing a patient's expressed need for help.

The basis of Orlando-Pelletier's Nursing Process theory consists of the three concepts of *patient behavior, nurse reaction that is explored with the patient,* and *nurse action* (George, 2002).

1. "The nursing process is set in motion by *patient behavior*. All patient behavior, no matter how insignificant, must be considered an expression of a need for help until its meaning to a particular patient in the immediate situation is understood. . . . Patient behavior may be verbal or nonverbal" (George, 2002, p. 193). Verbal behavior encompasses a patient's use of language, and nonverbal behavior includes physiologic symptoms, motor activity, and nonverbal communication. When a patient has a need for help that cannot be resolved without the help of another, helplessness results. If a patient's behavior does not effectively communicate an accurate depiction of the need for help, then difficulties in the nurse–patient relationship may arise and make it challenging for the nurse to adequately care for the patient. Resolution, or a clearer understanding of ineffective patient behavior, becomes a high priority for the nurse because the situation will likely worsen over time and make adequate care, or the provision of needed help, increasingly difficult. The nurse's actions and reactions are

designed to resolve ineffective patient behaviors and also meet the patient's immediate needs for help (George, 2002).

2. Patient behavior stimulates a *nurse reaction*, which is the start of the nursing process (Orlando, 1972). Appropriate nurse reaction consists of the following steps (George, 2002):

   - The nurse perceives the behavior through any of the senses.
   - The perception leads to an automatic thought.
   - The thought produces an automatic feeling.
   - The nurse shares reactions with the patient to ascertain whether perceptions are accurate or inaccurate.
   - The nurse consciously deliberates about personal reactions and patient input in order to produce professional deliberative actions based on mindful assessment rather than automatic reactions.

3. A nurse may act in one of two ways when providing care: automatic or deliberative. Professional *nursing actions* are nursing-care activities that result from deliberative activity on the part of the nurse rather than automatic reactions. Behaviors that stem from automatic rather than deliberative reactions do not meet the criteria for professional nursing behavior. Automatic reactions stem from nursing behaviors that are performed to satisfy a directive other than the patient's need for help. For example, the nurse who gives a sleeping pill to a patient every evening because it is ordered by the physician, without first discussing the need for the medication with the patient, is engaging in *automatic, nondeliberative* behavior. This is because the reason for giving the pill has more to do with following medical orders (automatically) than with the patient's immediate expressed need for help (George, 2002). The criteria for deliberative actions are as follows (George, 2002):

   - Deliberative actions result from the correct identification of patient needs by validation of the nurse's reaction to patient behavior.
   - The nurse explores the meaning of the action with the patient and its relevance to meeting the patient's need.
   - The nurse validates the action's effectiveness immediately after completing it.
   - The nurse is free of stimuli unrelated to the patient's need (when action is taken).

It can be argued that all nursing actions are meant to help the client and should be considered deliberative. However, for an action to have been truly deliberative, it must undergo reflective evaluation to determine whether the action helped the client by addressing a need as determined by the nurse and client in the immediate situation (George, 2002).

Assumptions that are inherent in Orlando-Pelletier's approach include the following (Tomey & Alligood, 2002):

- Nursing is allied with medicine and is also a distinct profession separate from other healthcare disciplines.
- Professional (deliberative) nursing has a distinct outcome product from other professions.
- The nurse's mind is the major helping tool.
- Each nurse–patient interaction is unique.
- The nurse's practice is improved by self-reflection.
- The nurse–patient interaction constitutes a dynamic whole.
- The actual nurse–patient encounter is a major source of nursing knowledge.
- Evidence of relieving distress is determined by the client's observable behavior.
- Promptly addressing a patient's need for help is important because the length of time a patient's needs go unmet influences the degree of distress.

Orlando (1990) aptly summarizes her theory as follows:

A deliberative nursing process has elements of continuous reflection as the nurse tries to understand the meaning to the patient of the behavior she observes and what he needs from her in order to be helped. Responses comprising this process are stimulated by the nurse's unfolding awareness of the particulars of the individual situation. (p. 67)

An origami design to express Orlando-Pelletier's Nursing Process theory would be a simple design with three large folds representing the three steps, or processes, of *patient behavior, nurse reaction,* and *nurse action.* Subsequent smaller folds would include the assumptions associated with the theory. The finished object might resemble a silhouette of two people connected to one another, alluding to the ongoing nurse and client interaction required for deliberative care to effectively take place.

Theory in Action

Nursing theories are meant to stimulate and support knowledge development related to effectively exploring, predicting, describing, defining, and (sometimes) controlling nursing phenomena. Orlando-Pelletier's Nursing Process theory is evident in how nurses function today. Nurse scholars have continued to develop and expand upon Nursing Process Theory. The two historical publications listed below, which are electronically accessible in the major databases, demonstrate Orlando-Pelletier's theory in action:

Schmieding, N. J. (1987). Action process of nurse administrators to problematic situations based on Orlando's theory. *Journal of Advanced Nursing*, 13, 99–107. doi:10.1111/j.1365-2648.1988.tb01396

This article presents a study that used Orlando-Pelletier's Nursing Process theory to explore how nurse administrators respond to problematic situations. Findings indicated that participants' first thoughts when a problem arose were seldom about staff response but rather focused on solving the problem alone or telling a staff member what to do to solve the problem.

Faust, C. (2002). Orlando's deliberative nursing process theory: A practice application in an extended care facility. *Journal of Gerontological Nursing*, 28(7), 14–18. doi:10.3928/0098-9134-20020701-05

This informational article sought to introduce Orlando-Pelletier's theory and demonstrate how it could be applied to nursing care in an extended care facility.

Learning Activities

Locate and read the two articles listed above to see how nurses have used Orlando-Pelletier's work.

1. Perform an Internet search using the word *origami* to view galleries of completed origami art. Choose one visual representation that depicts Orlando-Pelletier's theory and print a copy of it. Underneath the image, write a few sentences about why this particular origami creation depicts Orlando-Pelletier's theory. Share your picture with your classmates.

2. Find websites or journal articles on Orlando-Pelletier's theory. Words to use when performing a search might include:
   - Ida Jean Orlando-Pelletier
   - Nursing process
   - Nursing Process theory

References

George, J. B. (2002). *Nursing theories: The base for professional nursing practice.* Upper Saddle River, NJ: Prentice Hall.

Orlando, I. J. (1972). *The discipline and teaching of nursing process.* New York, NY: G. P. Putnam's Sons.

Orlando, I. J. (1990). *The dynamic nurse–patient relationship: Function, process, and principles.* New York, NY: National League for Nursing. (Reprinted from 1961, New York, NY: G. P. Putnam's Sons.)

Tomey, A. M., & Alligood, M. R. (2002). *Nursing theorists and their work* (5th ed.). St. Louis, MO: Mosby.

Katharine Kolcaba's Theory of Comfort

K atharine Kolcaba was born December 28, 1944, in Cleveland, Ohio. She received a diploma in nursing from St. Luke's Hospital School of Nursing in Cleveland. She then practiced for many years as a medical–surgical nurse, a long-term care nurse, and a homecare nurse. In 1987, Kolcaba graduated in the first RN to MSN class at Case Western Reserve University. While completing her master's degree, Kolcaba worked in a dementia unit, and it was there that she began theorizing about the concept of comfort. Upon completion of her MSN degree, Kolcaba became a faculty member at the University of Akron College of Nursing. Kolcaba received a doctorate in nursing in 1997 from Case Western Reserve and is certified in gerontology (Tomey & Alligood, 2002). She continues to teach and has published numerous articles discussing the concept of comfort as it relates to nursing. She has also published a book entitled *Comfort Theory and Practice: A Vision for Holistic Health Care and Research* (2003).

Kolcaba's Theory of Comfort specifically addresses the practice concept of nurse-provided comfort. It also describes a process by which comfort may be consistently delivered and evaluated by nurses. For these reasons, it is considered to be a middle-range theory.

Kolcaba's theory is based on the premise that one of most important nursing activities is that of providing comfort. The function of nursing, according to Kolcaba, is

> . . . the intentional assessment of comfort needs, design of comfort measures to address those needs, and reassessment of comfort levels after implementation compared to the previous baseline. Assessment and reassessment may be intuitive and/or subjective, such as when a nurse asks if the patient is comfortable, or objective, such as in observations of wound healing, changing lab values, or changes in behavior. Assessment can be achieved through the administration of visual analogue scales or traditional questionnaires. (Tomey & Alligood, 2002, p. 434)

The recipients of care may include individuals, family groups, institutions, or communities.

In a general sense, the term *comfort* could be defined as the experience of receiving effective care that meets comfort needs. There are three types of comfort and four contexts within which comfort occurs (Kolcaba, 1994). The three *types of comfort* defined by Kolcaba (1996) are the following:

1. *Relief* is the state of a patient who has had a specific need met.
2. *Ease* is a state of overall calm and contentment.
3. *Transcendence* is a state in which a person rises above problems and pain.

The experience of comfort occurs within different contexts. A desired result of appropriate comfort care would be optimal functioning in the following four contexts (Kolcaba, 1996):

1. *Physical* pertains to bodily sensations and homeostatic mechanisms.
2. *Psychospiritual* pertains to internal awareness of self, including esteem, sexuality, and life's meaning. It also includes a person's relationship to a higher being.
3. *Environmental* pertains to external surroundings, conditions, and influences. The environment may be altered by the patient, nurse, or others to enhance comfort.
4. *Sociocultural* pertains to interpersonal, family, and societal relationships, as well as family traditions, rituals, and religious practices.

Nurses provide comfort through *comfort measures* that are designed to meet the needs of individual patients. Comfort needs may be associated with physical, psychospiritual, environmental, or sociocultural factors (Kolcaba, 1994). Comfort needs are expressed by the patient and assessed by the nurse through nurse monitoring of verbal or nonverbal reports, pathophysiologic parameters, education deficits, need for support, and financial stresses. *Intervening variables*, which are factors that influence a patient's perception of total comfort, might include past experiences, age, attitude, emotional state, support system, prognosis, and finances. The specific combinations of the number and types of *comfort measures needed*, *context*, and *intervening variables* influence a patient's overall perception of the level and type of comfort experienced.

Four broad assumptions and theoretical assertions that help form the basis of Kolcaba's work are listed here. Knowledge of these assumptions clarifies the meaning of the theory (Kolcaba, 1994):

- Human beings have wholistic responses to complex stimuli.
- Comfort is a wholistic outcome of effective nursing care.
- Human beings have a need for comfort and will seek comfort wherever possible.
- Nurses are in a position to identify the comfort needs of their patients, design comfort measures, and assess outcomes to support enhanced comfort.

In summary, the presence or absence of patient comfort is an often-addressed issue in nursing practice. Kolcaba's Theory of Comfort lends structure and meaning to the term *comfort* as it applies to the nurse–patient relationship. Kolcaba (1994) stated, "The understanding of comfort directly guides nursing care that is inclusive of physical, psychospiritual, social and environmental interventions.... Clinicians have the capability and disciplinary interest to effect comfort, and patients look to nurses for help in achieving comfort" (p. 1183). Exploration and explanation of this often-used concept will allow nurses to formally study the phenomenon of comfort and discern care practices that support optimal patient comfort.

An origami design that might express Kolcaba's Theory of Comfort would consist of seven folds representing the three levels of comfort (*relief*, *ease*, and *transcendence*) and the four contexts in which comfort occurs (*physical*, *psychospiritual*, *environmental*, and *sociocultural*). The finished object would resemble a patchwork quilt, representing the *comfort* one might experience when wrapped up in a warm handmade quilt on a rainy day.

Reflections About Comfort Theory

Kathy Kolcaba

Some of you know that I wrote *Comfort Theory* (CT) because it was required for my dissertation. Specifically, a theory was required to underpin my mandatory comfort study and thus required for graduation. My dilemma was that there were no nursing theories that remotely referred to patient comfort, so I looked at earlier nursing dissertations for any existing theory that would have the following criteria: it had to have a high level of abstraction (so I could link comfort into it), it had to be centered on patients (because ideas were related to their comfort needs), and it had to have adequate explanatory power (so I could learn something from it). Lo and behold, I found Edward Murray's framework from the 1930s, recently used by a graduate of our program, and I was able to link comfort and other nursing concepts beneath his original generic ones. My lower theoretical level was more concrete and specific to health care than Murray's, and I called that level my mid-range theory of comfort. I was able to place comfort, which needed a home, right at the heart of it all.

My newly formulated theory served nicely for my dissertation study, but when I told my advisor I wanted to try to publish it before my dissertation was completed (another 2–3 years), she balked. She didn't want me to take the time to do this—but I did it anyway, quietly, and CT was published about a year later. This style of being a theorist became the norm for me, in that my ideas did not come out of thin air; they were initiated by external forces beyond my control, they were controlled by institutional politics, and they were not given enthusiastic support at first. I did not let myself be deterred when my theoretical work was rejected for conference presentations. Even though I did not yet have data to support CT, I stubbornly believed that this idea of comfort should be central to nursing much as it was at the beginning of our profession. Indeed, perhaps comfort is needed even more in modern nursing, as an antidote to all the high-tech equipment. Also, my zodiac sign is Capricorn, and I always thought that the goat was a good description of how I plodded along toward my goal of broad acceptance of CT, going around or over hurdles by finding greener pastures *somewhere*, all the while making modest headway by putting one foot in front of the other.

Another important factor for me was that, as a teacher, I had the discretion of imposing CT on my own students and observing what worked and didn't work for them and their patients. What I saw was that the students enjoyed intentionally comforting their patients in many technical and not-so-technical ways and (yes . . .) including all of these ways on their daily comfort care plans. Unlike the usual sterile nursing process format, comfort care plans required that students record everything they did for their patients, including such comforting interventions as repositioning, rubbing patients' backs, walking and talking with them, cleaning up their rooms, etc. Because comfort care plans are holistic, students could record their interventions in no particular order after they identified individual comfort needs, and they could record their patients' responses to these interventions. This sort of documentation then provided a very complete and unique picture of each patient. Of course, the patients loved all this attention to their comfort, too. And together, through positive and negative feedback from students and patients, CT became richer, more relevant, and more useful. For example, students questioned me about the lack of emphasis on physiological problems in CT, so I saw that I needed to strengthen my definition of physical comfort. They asked, "Who cares about patient comfort besides the patient?" and I added the concept of institutional integrity to the model. For the advancement of CT, this sort of feedback was and is invaluable to me. So valuable, in fact, that I continue to teach my theory course in the summer, even though I am otherwise retired from the University of Akron after teaching full time for 22 years.

While waiting for my wannabe presentations to be more widely heard, my theory to be published in nursing textbooks, and nursing politics to discover that comfort is an outcome that patients and families want and need, I was adding students' ideas and observations about patients who were comforted to my Web site. Because updating could occur quickly on the Web, this became my preferred venue for modifying CT and for building my network with like-minded students and nurses. Come visit me in cyberspace at www.thecomfortline.com.

When Magnet status was created to reward nurse-friendly hospitals, I saw an opportunity to take my theory on the road. The Magnet award gave a big boost to nursing theory in general because the criteria for Magnet were many, expensive, and difficult to achieve, requiring that all nurses and administrators in a given hospital be on the same page. This was much easier if nurses utilized a theory for focus. CT was particularly pertinent because nurses could use it to improve their working environment, so I redefined the four contexts of comfort in terms of nurses' comfort. Nurses loved being asked, first by me and then by their bosses, for their comfort wish lists—ideas that would turn their workplaces into comfort zones.

I never intended to be an entrepreneur, but I began my business called *The Comfort Line* (named after my Web site) as a way to promote nursing, specifically the *art* of nursing in which nurses comfort their patients and families in many creative, satisfying ways. Even though most nurses were doing this intuitively, modern charting provided no place to report comfort work, and so it was undervalued by administrators and underrecognized by the general public.

Therefore, when introducing CT to a new class or audience, I often ask for personal experiences if they or a family member had been recipients of nursing that made a difference. Their stories (I call them "memorable nurse" stories) show how meaningful those nursing acts of compassion and comforting are for healing. Usually, nurses who comforted them were the only ones the students remembered.

Why was comfort important for healing? The original meaning of comfort, or *confortare*, is "to strengthen greatly." I refer to this meaning frequently to propose that patients who are comforted do better in surgical healing, therapies, and learning new regimens for health and discharge planning (health-seeking behaviors). This made administrators interested, because their financial bottom line (or institutional integrity) could be improved. With nurse leaders, I also suggested that institutions that adopted CT for their practice framework would find that their nurses would be more productive (remember the comfort wish lists), better able to comfort and strengthen their patients, and more likely to stay in that hospital system because their work was satisfying and visible.

Recently, patient satisfaction became an important national and public measuring stick for how hospitals compare with others. So I again adapted CT to this trend. In this way, I found that, if I kept on top of the trends, I could adapt CT to fit most innovations or needs in health care today. I could also instantly adapt the material on my Web site and make it and myself available through new and nifty technologies that students and many practicing nurses would value, such as podcasts and webcasts. Getting patient comfort accepted politically remains my most difficult challenge—gatekeepers at the highest levels of nursing are frustratingly inaccessible and/or closed to ideas outside their boxes.

I had many lucky stars that lined up to guide my way and support me when I got tired or discouraged. These stars include my graduate programs and professors at Case Western Reserve University, my students at the University of Akron, my family, my research team members, nurses in my consulting hospitals, and the patients and families who demonstrated the significance of comforting interventions in ways large and profound. All of these stars enabled this old goat to plod along toward the next adaptation and application of CT. (Actually, at this writing, I am a very spry and adventuresome 64 years.) I hope that you will all consider being future guiding lights for comfort theory. Thank you, one and all!

Theory in Action

Nursing theories are meant to stimulate and support knowledge development related to effectively exploring, predicting, describing, defining, and (sometimes) controlling nursing phenomena. Kolcaba's work is groundbreaking in that she created a theory to facilitate deepened understanding of a common, yet critical concept that is often unexamined because it is considered a by-product of good nursing care rather than end in itself. The two publications listed below, which are electronically accessible in the major databases, demonstrate Kolcaba's theory in action:

March, A., & McCormack, D. (2009). Modifying Kolcaba's Comfort Theory as an institution-wide approach. *Holistic Nursing Practice*, 23(2), 75–80. doi:10.1097/HNP.0b013e3181a1105b

The authors of this article discuss how slightly modifying Kolcaba's Comfort Theory could facilitate its interdisciplinary use to support continuity of care within one institution.

Krinsky, R., Murillo, I., & Johnson, J. (2014). A practical application of Katharine Kolcaba's Comfort Theory to cardiac patients. *Applied Nursing Research*, 27, 147–150. doi:org/10.1016/j.apnr.2014.02.004

In this article, Kolcaba's Comfort Theory is applied to cardiac nursing. The specific intervention of "quiet time" is described as a potential intervention for patients who are suffering from multiple symptoms from cardiac syndromes.

Learning Activities

Locate and read the two articles listed above to see how nurses have used Kolcaba's work.

1. Perform an Internet search using the word *origami* to view galleries of completed origami art. Choose one visual representation that depicts Kolcaba's theory and print a copy of it. Underneath the image, write a few sentences about how this particular origami creation depicts Kolcaba's theory. Share the project with classmates.
2. Find websites or journal articles about Kolcaba's theory. Words to use when performing a search might include:
   • Katharine Kolcaba
   • Comfort
   • Comfort care
   • Theory of Comfort care

References

Kolcaba, K. (1994). A theory of holistic comfort for nursing. *Journal of Advanced Nursing*, 19, 1178–1184.

Kolcaba, K. (1996). A holistic perspective on comfort care as an advance directive. *Critical Care Nursing Quarterly*, 18(4), 66–79.

Kolcaba, K. (2003). Comfort theory and practice: A vision for holistic health care and research. New York, NY: Springer-Verlag.

Tomey, A. M., & Alligood, M. R. (2002). *Nursing theorists and their work* (5th ed.). St. Louis, MO: Mosby.

Nola Pender's Health-Promotion Model

Nola Pender was born in Lansing, Michigan, in 1941. She was an only child, and her parents were advocates for the education of women. At the age of 7, Pender took note of the nursing care her hospitalized aunt received, and this prompted an early interest in nursing. Further education strengthened her interest in obtaining a nursing degree, and with family support, Pender received her diploma from the School of Nursing at West Suburban Hospital in Oak Park, Illinois, in 1962. She then worked in medical–surgical and pediatric nursing. She completed a Bachelor of Science in nursing at Michigan State University in East Lansing in 1964. In 1965, Pender earned a Master of Arts degree in human growth and development from Michigan State University and in 1969 completed a doctorate in psychology and education at Northwestern University in Evanston, Illinois. Several years after completing her doctorate, Pender completed master's-level studies in community health nursing at Rush University in Chicago. Since 1990, Pender has been professor and associate dean for research at the University of Michigan School of Nursing. Pender has published many articles about exercise, behavior change, and relaxation training and has edited many journals and books. The fifth edition of her book on her Health Promotion Model was published in 2006.

Pender (2003) explains the importance of health promotion as follows:

> Very early in my nursing career, it became apparent to me that health professionals intervened only after people developed acute or chronic disease and experienced compromised lives. Attention was devoted to treating them after the fact. This reactive approach did not reflect the philosophical beliefs of our predecessors in nursing who focused on maintaining conditions of a healthy interaction between self and the environment. . . . I committed myself to the proactive stance of health promotion and disease prevention with the conviction that it is much better to experience exuberant well-being and prevent disease than let disease happen when it is avoidable and then try and cope with it.

Health-promoting behaviors are a desired outcome when providing client care and education. Health-promoting behaviors may be defined as an action directed toward attaining positive health outcomes such as optimal well-being, personal fulfillment, and productive living (Tomey & Alligood, 2002). Examples of health-promoting behaviors include eating a healthy diet, exercising regularly, managing stress, gaining adequate rest, enhancing spiritual growth, and building positive relationships. Nurses in all practice areas have numerous opportunities to encourage health-promoting behaviors related to presenting concerns and anticipated health challenges. Pender (1996) identifies the following factors as having a potential influence on the health-promoting behaviors of clients. Whereas the first two items on the list (prior related behavior and personal factors) are difficult (or impossible) for a nurse to change, the other factors listed can be influenced positively by nurses through effective assessment, support, and education. Pender's (1996) factors include the following:

- *Prior related behavior* refers to the past frequency of behaviors. The more frequently a behavior was done in the past, the more likely it is that the behavior will continue in the future.
- *Personal factors* include biological, psychological, and sociocultural factors that directly and indirectly influence health-promoting behaviors.
  - *Biological factors* include age, gender, body mass index, onset of puberty or menopause, aerobic capacity, strength, agility, and balance.
  - *Psychological factors* include self-esteem, self-motivation, personal competence, perceived health status, and individual definition of health.
  - *Sociocultural factors* include race, ethnicity, cultural identity within the larger culture, educational opportunities, and socioeconomic status.

- *Perceived benefits of action* are the expected positive outcomes of the proposed health-promoting behavior. For example, a teenager may be prompted to quit smoking after the nurse comments that smoking causes teeth to become discolored and that after quitting teeth will remain whiter and healthier.
- *Perceived barriers to action* are the real and imagined barriers to health behavior change. For example, financial limitations might make it impossible for a client to maintain a membership at a gym (a real barrier). Another client may be able to pay for the gym membership only to be thwarted by an imagined barrier such as, "Everyone will laugh and stare at me every time I go to the gym because I am not in good physical condition."
- *Perceived self-efficacy* refers to personal judgment about individual capability to organize and consistently perform new behaviors. Higher self-efficacy results in lowered perceptions of possible barriers to positive health behavior change. For example, if a person perceives himself or herself as being well organized and motivated toward self-betterment, that person is less likely to encounter significant barriers to behavioral change than someone who feels disorganized and unmotivated.
- *Activity-related effect* refers to negative and positive behaviors associated with actually doing the health-promoting behavior. For example, if a person resolves to walk a mile during lunch break every day at work and finds that the result is fatigue and unpleasantly sweaty work clothes, then the feelings associated with the actual activity of walking for fitness at work may be negative.
- *Interpersonal influences* refer to how the significant others around the client affect motivation for positive change. These influences include expectations, social support, and modeling by family, peers, and healthcare providers. If a client lives in a household where all the adults smoke, then smoking cessation will be more difficult than if the client is the only adult who smokes and the rest of the family would prefer for the client to quit.
- *Situational influences* refer to external factors that affect the client's perception of the proposed health-promoting behavior, such as where, when, and how the activity will take place. For example, if a client is asked to attend a nutrition education class in the lobby of a candy store, the smell and inviting appearance of the candy might make it impossible for the client to commit to a weight loss program unless the competing demand of the irresistible candy is removed.

- *Commitment to a plan of action* refers to the person's intention to change and the creation of a plan of action to accomplish the implementation of a health-promoting behavior. Clients are more likely to engage in health-promoting behaviors when they anticipate realizing specific benefits from the activity.
- *Immediate competing demands* are behaviors over which the client has little control because they are associated with necessary life activities, such as work or family care responsibilities. For example, if a client had to choose between leaving a child home alone to go to the gym or staying home with the child, most parents would choose to stay home rather than leave the child alone. In this situation, exploring exercise options that would include time spent with the child may be more effective in the long run than attempting to complete an exercise regime at a gym.
- *Competing preferences* are those choices over which a client has a high degree of control, such as whether to eat an apple or a candy bar for an afternoon snack. Education regarding healthy rather than poor food choices would enable the client to adjust personal preferences and make better-informed decisions that would support healthy eating behaviors.

Knowledge of the assumptions that form the foundation of a theory are helpful in clarifying the overall thrust and meaning of the theory. Pender's Health Promotion Model is based on the following assumptions (Pender, 2003; Pender, Murdaugh, & Parsons, 2002):

- Individuals seek to create conditions of living through which they can express their unique human potential.
- Individuals have the capacity for reflective self-awareness, including assessment of their own competencies.
- Individuals value growth in directions viewed as positive and attempt to achieve a personally acceptable balance between change and stability.
- Individuals seek to actively regulate their own behavior.
- Individuals in all their biopsychosocial complexity interact with the environment, progressively transforming the environment and themselves over time.

- Health professionals constitute a part of the interpersonal environment, which exerts influence on persons throughout their life span.
- Self-initiated reconfiguration of person–environment interactive patterns is essential to behavior change.

Many nurse theorists create diagrams or abstract visual representations of theory concepts. Most of these creations require comprehensive knowledge and understanding of a theory before they can be fully appreciated or understood. Because Pender's model is relatively simple and self-explanatory, it is included here (see **Figure 19.1**).

In summary, Pender's Health Promotion Model proposes a structured process for assessing and addressing client needs associated with healthy behaviors. This model is based on combined nursing and behavioral health approaches that are meant to help clients make positive health behavioral changes. Pender's model provides immediately applicable principles to help nurses systematically address this important issue. Nurses who are aware of

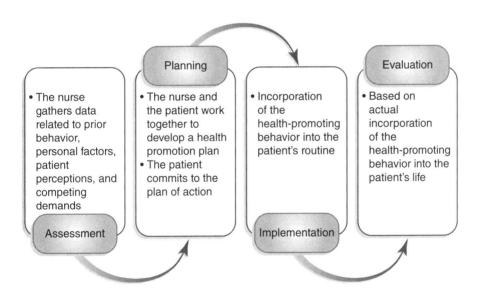

Figure 19.1 Pender's Health Promotion Model.

specific concerns related to promoting healthy behavior are more effective in supporting long-term positive health behaviors and activities for all clients.

An origami design to express Pender's Health Promotion Model might be a simple design depicting an apple (remember the old saying, "An apple a day keeps the doctor away"?). The first two folds of the design would represent *prior related behavior* and *personal factors*. Subsequent folds would incorporate the factors that nurses are able to assist clients in changing, such as *perceived benefits, perceived barriers, self-efficacy, activity-related effect, interpersonal influences, situational influences,* and *immediate competing demands*. The last fold would represent a *commitment to a plan of action*. The final result of all of these folds would be an apple representing health-promoting behaviors.

The Adventures of a Nurse Theorist

Nola J. Pender

I am excited to share with you my lifelong adventure in helping nurses develop knowledge and skills in the areas of prevention and health promotion. As you read my personal narrative, I hope you will consider what new insights, ideas, or theory you can contribute to nursing to improve our profession. I know that every nurse has the potential for creative work because I hear endless fascinating ideas in conversations with nurses. Getting our ideas out of our heads and on paper for others to benefit from is a challenge. However, once you take a deep breath and plunge ahead to meet that challenge, your work has the potential for altering nursing forever and contributing to the development of our beloved profession.

The Beginning

A man thrashes in his bed as his chest pain strikes again. He looks at me with anxious eyes. Please help, his eyes plead. Suddenly the pain strikes again, and he cries, "I am going to die! I am going to die!"

A woman who is diabetic and markedly overweight is trying to work out at the fitness center at the hospital. She looks at me, perspiring profusely and trying to get her breath. "I just can't do this, I just can't do this," she gasps. "Why did I ever let myself get in this shape?"

A small child looks up at me with sad eyes. She was playing with matches at home and her clothes caught on fire. She knows that today her bandages will need to be changed and she is gripped with fear.

These are the images that I encountered as I worked as a nurse in medical–surgical and pediatric settings. I began to wonder why nurses could not *prevent* such tragic human situations. All this suffering might have been prevented with healthy lifestyles and healthy environments.

As I pursued my graduate education, I began to read about wellness. Halbert Dunn wrote about high-level wellness. John Travis wrote about a wellness lifestyle. I asked myself, was high-level wellness wishful thinking or was it really attainable? Then I had that aha moment—helping people achieve the highest level of health or wellness possible to maximize quality of life is what nursing is all about. Wellness is the goal of nursing as Florence Nightingale intended it to be. Wellness and health promotion needed much more attention in nursing!

Family members play a crucial role in the direction our life takes. In my case, my husband, who had just completed his doctorate, urged me to go on for doctoral work. His support was crucial in the next phase of my life as a budding theorist. I pursued a doctoral degree at Northwestern University with a dual major in education and psychology. The more immersed I became in learning about how people think and make decisions, the more motivated I became to combine nursing and psychology to create a model to help nurses understand how people can change their thinking and behavior to adopt healthy lifestyles. I was excited, motivated, and having fun trying to organize my thoughts about critical aspects of health counseling by nurses.

Along the Way

After I finished my doctoral degree, I accepted my first teaching position at Northern Illinois University. After I taught for 3 years, we had our first child, a daughter. The next year we had our son. Two wonderful children! As I looked into their eyes, I was even more motivated to move nursing in the direction of health promotion. If we could create healthy lifestyles for children by working with them and their families, then healthy living would unfold early in life and hopefully carry forward into adulthood. Being a mother was a continuing source of motivation to make a difference in nursing, for the sake of my children and thousands of children worldwide.

People are our inspiration at each step in life. I had very special colleagues at Northern Illinois University. Dr. Beverly McElmurry inspired me with her interest in health as the focus for nursing curricula. Drs. Susan Walker, Karen Sechrist, and Marilyn Stromborg and I began discussions about the role of nurses in promoting healthy living. By that time, I had drafted a health promotion model (HPM) that combined ideas from nursing, education, and psychology about the trigger points for promoting health behavior change. My colleagues and I decided to apply for research monies to test the model and see if it worked. We were funded for a total of 5 years of research to test the HPM with adults. The model did predict health behaviors, but after looking at the research findings carefully, we decided that a model that had behavior-specific variables might be even more predictive and helpful. Thus, after our discussion, the health promotion model was revised. For example, rather than focusing on self-esteem, we adopted Dr. Albert Bandura's concept of self-efficacy or confidence in ability to perform a specific behavior. Other changes were made also. A model or theory evolves as research findings indicate how to improve it. Ideas that spring from our heads or that we adapt from another field are just that—ideas—they need to be tested; that is what we accomplish through our research.

After I moved to the University of Michigan, further funding for research allowed me to test the HPM with children and physical activity. The model did have some predictive power, which was encouraging. Other colleagues at the University of Michigan were also testing the model. Dr. Sally Lusk and her colleagues developed an extensive research program testing the HPM with adults in regard to hearing protection and conservation. It was encouraging to see that an intervention based on the HPM did increase worker use of hearing protection.

The next adventure in testing the HPM was a funded pilot study conducted with Dr. Lorraine Robbins and Dr. Kimberlee Gretebeck to test a nurse practitioner counseling intervention to increase physical activity among middle school girls. With this pilot intervention, we saw changes in beliefs, but we did not see significant changes in physical activity. That was a disappointment. However, not easily discouraged, we went back to the drawing board to see what we could do to increase the impact of the intervention. Currently, Dr. Robbins is funded to test the enhanced intervention with adolescent girls from diverse cultures. The results of her study will determine if the behavioral counseling intervention for adolescent girls, based on the HPM, really does improve their level of physical activity.

In addition to the aforementioned studies, many other research studies, including dissertations, have been conducted using the HPM. It is fun to get e-mails almost every day from students asking for further information about the model or telling me about their work with the model.

Looking Ahead

I am very fortunate to have made a contribution to nurses' awareness of the importance of health promotion and to their knowledge and ability to counsel patients for lifestyle change. However, theories and models are not created in a vacuum. Many people motivate and inspire us along the way. Our patients, our families, our coworkers, and the writings of professionals who have gone before us all fuel our interest, our thoughts, and our passion for creative work in nursing. In my case, the spark for a lifelong career came from seeing patients in distress whose distress might have been prevented through healthy living. Your spark may be another life-changing clinical experience.

As the science for evidence-based practice continues to evolve, the profession of nursing needs new models and theories. New theories that are better than older ones emerge, and the new theories replace theories from the past. That is the natural evolution of knowledge in nursing. By being alert to your clinical environment, listening to your patients and colleagues, and playing with clinical ideas in new combinations, you, too, can become a nurse theorist. We need your contribution to nursing, both now and for the future. Remember, for theories to be of value to nursing, they must be useful. They must help us with our everyday interactions with patients. Theories or models that begin in nursing interactions and nursing observations are most likely to serve nursing well as we continue to develop as a caring science. Join the adventure!

Theory in Action

Nursing theories are meant to stimulate and support knowledge development related to effectively exploring, predicting, describing, defining, and (sometimes) controlling nursing phenomena. Pender's work was groundbreaking in that she was the first nurse to fully create and extensively develop a health promotion model specifically related to nursing. Pender demonstrated great foresight. Health promotion has become a major focus of nursing care in the twenty-first century. The two publications listed below, which are electronically accessible in the major databases, demonstrate Pender's theory in action:

McCullaugh, M., Lusk, S. L., & Ronis, D. L. (2002). Factors influencing use of hearing protection among farmers: A test of the Pender Health Promotion Model. *Nursing Research*, 51(1), 33–39. doi:10.1097/00006199-200201000-00006

This article presents a study that utilized Pender's Health Promotion Model to identify factors that affected farmers' use of hearing protection. Results showed that interpersonal support, barriers, and situational factors predicted whether hearing protection would be used.

Ho, A. Y. K. , Berggren, I., & Dahlborg-Lyckhage, E. (2010). Diabetes empowerment related to Pender's Health Promotion Model: A meta-synthesis. *Nursing and Health Sciences*, 12, 259–267. doi:10.1111/j.1442-2018.2010.00517.x

In this meta-synthesis, nine qualitative studies were assessed to determine effective empowerment strategies for diabetes self-management. Based on Pender's Health Promotion Model, the authors asserted that healthcare professionals must assess and work with behavior-specific variables to support health-promoting behaviors.

Learning Activities

Locate and read the two articles listed above to see how nurses have used Pender's work.

1. Perform an Internet search using the word *origami* to view galleries of completed origami art. Choose one visual representation that depicts Pender's model and print a copy of it. Underneath the image, write a few sentences about how this particular origami creation depicts Pender's model. Share your project with your classmates.
2. Find websites or journal articles about Pender's model. Words to use when performing a search might include:
   - Nola Pender
   - Health promotion
   - Health Promotion Model

References

Pender, N. J. (1996). *Health promotion in nursing practice* (3rd ed.). Stamford, CT: Appleton & Lange.

Pender, N. J. (2003). Frequent questions. Retrieved from http://www.nursing.umich.edu/faculty/pender/pender_questions.html

Pender, N. J., Murdaugh, C. L., & Parsons, M. A. (2002). *Health promotion in nursing practice* (4th ed.). Upper Saddle River, NJ: Prentice Hall.

Tomey, A. M., & Alligood, M. R. (2002). *Nursing theorists and their work* (5th ed.). St. Louis, MO: Mosby.

Hildegard Peplau's Interpersonal Relations in Nursing

Hildegard Peplau was born in Reading, Pennsylvania, in 1909. In 1931, Peplau graduated from the Pennsylvania School of Nursing and began her nursing career. She earned a Bachelor of Arts degree in interpersonal psychology from Bennington College, Vermont. Peplau also completed a Master of Arts degree in psychiatric nursing in 1947 and a Doctor of Education degree in curriculum development in 1953 at Teachers College at Columbia University. Peplau taught graduate psychiatric nursing at Columbia University and then taught at Rutgers University for 20 years, earning the title of Professor Emeritus. Peplau died peacefully in Sherman Oaks, California, in 1999.

During her long career, Peplau contributed greatly to the development of psychiatric nursing and to the advancement of nursing as a profession. In 1952, Peplau's book *Interpersonal Relations in Nursing* described the relationship between nurse and client. Peplau is considered a visionary because she published this work during a time when the creation of nursing theories was not a focal point in the profession (George, 2002). Many believe that this book caused a shift in perception from the accepted practice of the nurse performing interventions *on or to* a patient to the nurse and patient acting in partnership during the care process (Tomey & Alligood, 2002).

Peplau (1988) broadly describes nursing as

> . . .a significant, therapeutic, interpersonal process. It functions coop-
> eratively with other human processes that make health possible for
> individuals in communities. . . . Nursing is an educative instrument, a
> maturing force that aims to promote forward movement of personality
> in the direction of creative, constructive, productive, personal, and
> community living. (p. 16)

Understanding and applying Peplau's theory first requires participant
observations by the nurse in three focal areas. The nurse must consciously
observe

1. His or her own behaviors
2. The behaviors demonstrated by the patient
3. The type and quality of relations that occur between nurse and patient

This calls for honest, and sometimes uncomfortable, self-appraisal by the
nurse that is meant to ultimately result in the nurse becoming more aware of
what messages are being communicated to the patient (Peplau, 1997). Gaining
a better understanding helps the nurse avoid interpersonal pitfalls within the
nurse–patient exchange, such as (Peplau, 1997):

- Labeling the patient, either intentionally or unintentionally
- Comparing the patient with others
- Competing with the patient by trying to "one-up" them in some way
- Taking advantage of the patient by using care time to talk about the
  nurse's personal experiences rather than the patient's
- Expecting the patient to change after one nurse–patient interaction
- Declining to discuss difficult or emotional topics with the patient
- Avoiding patients rather than honestly addressing anger or annoyance

Peplau describes multiple roles that the nurse may fulfill within a nurse–
patient relationship. These roles are best managed if the nurse actively
observes and appraises self, patient, and the quality of relations on an ongoing basis. Some of the roles include (Peplau, 1952, 1988):

- Stranger
- Teacher

- Healthcare resource person
- Leader
- Counselor
- Safety agent
- Mediator
- Observer

The nurse may fulfill many roles in addition to those just listed when providing care to individuals. Enactment of a role should depend on the need of the patient at any given time. Through careful observation, nurses are able to choose what role might fit best within specific situations to support optimal patient outcomes.

Peplau (1997) described three overlapping phases representing the structure of the nurse–patient relationship:

1. *The orientation phase* is when the nurse and patient are getting acquainted with one another. This is when the nurse clarifies what she or he will do within the nurse–patient relationship. It is also when the nurse gains information on what the patient wants and expects from the relationship. Active listening on the part of the nurse is especially important during this phase (although listening is important in all phases).
2. *The working phase* is when most of the pointed and intense interaction occurs and is also when the nurse is likely to assume multiple roles in the relationship as needed in order to help the patient experience a positive outcome. Through self-evaluation and careful observation, nurses may professionally mature during the working phase through increasing understanding of how and why they relate to individual patients in certain ways.
3. *The termination phase* is when nurses and patients summarize the work accomplished and move toward closure of the relationship. Discharge planning is usually initiated prior to starting the termination phase so that patients have an opportunity to gradually move toward termination rather than experience an abrupt transition at the end of care.

In summary, Peplau's *Interpersonal Relations in Nursing* describes a basic framework within which nurses and patients interact. Because it describes one component of nursing care (the interaction between patient and nurse), it is a middle-range theory. However, the basic nature of this theory allows for its application by every nurse in a wide range of situations. This theory is profoundly important because it was the first to propose that instead of *doing things to* a patient, a nurse must *provide care in partnership with* the patient.

An origami design to express Peplau's Interpersonal Relations in Nursing theory might be a design consisting of three different colors of paper: one representing the patient, one representing the nurse, and one representing the relationship. The three papers are intertwined into the form of a triangle with three sides, each side made up of all three colors. The completed triangle represents the completed relationship, consisting of the three sides, or steps, of the relationship: the orientation phase, the working phase, and the termination phase. The symmetry and form of the design symbolize the positive and satisfying interpersonal exchange that results for both the nurse and the patient when the nurse consciously employs the concepts described by Peplau.

Theory in Action

Nursing theories are meant to stimulate and support knowledge development related to effectively exploring, predicting, describing, defining, and (sometimes) controlling nursing phenomena. Peplau's work was visionary in that she sought to describe the nurse–patient relationship within a collaborative framework, making the patient and nurse partners in care, healing, and wellness. The two publications listed below, which are electronically accessible in the major databases, demonstrate Peplau's theory in action:

Senn, J. F. (2013). Peplau's theory of interpersonal relations: Application in emergency and rural nursing. *Nursing Science Quarterly*, 26, 31–35. doi:10.1177/0894318412466744

This application to practice article discusses Peplau's Theory of Interpersonal Relations in relation to emergency nursing and rural nursing. The authors conclude that skillful nurse–patient interactions in both settings rest on communication patterns that mirror those described by Peplau.

Delaney, K. R., & Ferguson, J. (2014). Peplau and the brain: Why interpersonal neuroscience provides a useful language for the relationship process. *Journal of Nursing Education and Practice*, 4(8), 145–152. doi:10.5430/jnep.v4n8p145

The authors of this article discuss the significant impact of Peplau's work in relation to psychiatric mental health (PMH) nursing and propose reexamination of the therapeutic relationship model in relation to current PMH practices. The authors expand on Peplau's model to create a neuroscience engagement process meant to promote healing in mental health patients.

Learning Activities

Locate and read the two articles listed above to see how nurses have used Peplau's work.

1. Perform an Internet search using the word *origami* to view galleries of completed origami art. Choose one visual representation that depicts Peplau's model and print a copy of it. Underneath the image, write a few sentences about how this particular origami creation depicts Peplau's model. Share your project with your classmates.
2. Find websites or journal articles on Peplau's theory. Words to use when performing a search might include:
   - Hildegard Peplau
   - Interpersonal Relations in Nursing

References

George, J. B. (2002). *Nursing theories: The base for professional nursing practice*. Upper Saddle River, NJ: Prentice Hall.

Peplau, H. E. (1952). *Interpersonal relations in nursing*. New York, NY: G. P. Putnam's Sons.

Peplau, H. E. (1988). *Interpersonal relations in nursing*. London, England: Macmillan Press Limited.

Peplau, H. E. (1997). Peplau's theory of interpersonal relations. *Nursing Science Quarterly*, 10(4), 162–167.

Tomey, A. M., & Alligood, M. R. (2002). *Nursing theorists and their work* (5th ed.). St. Louis, MO: Mosby.

Imogene King's Conceptual System and Theory of Goal Attainment

I mogene M. King, who developed the Theory of Goal Attainment, was born on January 30, 1923, in West Point, Iowa. King earned a diploma in nursing from St. John's Hospital School of Nursing in St. Louis, Missouri, in 1945, and Bachelor and Master of Science degrees in nursing from St. Louis University in 1948 and 1957, respectively. King worked as an instructor and assistant director at the St. John's Hospital School of Nursing from 1947 until 1958 while working on her bachelor's and master's degrees. King studied under Mildred Montag, creator of associate degree nursing at Teachers College, Columbia University, earning her Master of Education degree in 1961 (Messmer, 2000).

After receiving her doctorate degree, Dr. King worked as an associate professor of nursing at Loyola University, where she began publishing her work on nursing theory (Tomey & Alligood, 2006). King served as the assistant chief of the Research Grants Branch, Division of Nursing, in Washington, D.C., from 1966 to 1968 under Dr. Jessie M. Scott. From 1968 to 1972, King was director and professor in the school of nursing at The Ohio State University. Her book, *Toward a Theory for Nursing: General Concepts of Human Behavior* (King, 1971), was published during her tenure at Ohio State. In 1972, King returned to Loyola University, where she coordinated clinical research in the School of Nursing until 1980, when she moved to the University of South Florida in Tampa as a professor of nursing. She worked at South Florida until her retirement in 1990. After her retirement, she continued to work with the King International Nursing Group (KING) to advance her theory. King, a Sigma Theta Tau International Virginia Henderson fellow, was a recipient of the Elizabeth Russell Belford Founders Award for Excellence in Education. In 1994, she was inducted into the American Academy of Nursing and, in 1996, received the Jessie M. Scott Award from the American Nurses Association.

King enjoyed eclectic interests, including abstract painting, golf, politics, and daytime soap operas (Messmer, 2009). King gave generously of her time to help students better understand her theory, allowing her email address to be published on Eichelberger's Nursing Theory website. She communicated daily with students and others interested in her theory. However, she was adamant that a website on her theory not be created. Members of KING were working on a KING website when King asked that they stop. She appeared to be uncomfortable with the Web and concerned that her work would be misrepresented (Bev Whelan, personal communication, April 20, 2008). She never married and died at the age of 84 on Christmas Eve, 2007, in Florida. King's papers and memorabilia are at Loyola University in Chicago, Illinois.

Conceptual System

In 1971, King wrote her first textbook, which outlined a conceptual framework, later called a conceptual system, that nurses could use to identify and analyze nursing situations. King's framework was a "way of thinking about the real world of nursing" (King, 1971, p. 125). She also outlined the process of developing theory as either inductive or deductive, where one could develop a theory and then test it in practice through research or develop theory deduced from research data. King stated that both methods had value.

King's work is considered a conceptual model by some because it encompasses both a conceptual framework and a theory (King, 2001). King's conceptual view of nursing is based on Von Bertanlanffy's general systems theory, which influenced her to study the complexity of nursing by identifying *Imogene King—Conceptual System and Theory of Goal Attainment* and analyzing the interdependent variables and concepts that exist in phenomena (King, 2007). King defined a system as a set of components linked by communication that exhibit directed behaviors for the purpose of attaining goals, thus giving rise to her Theory of Goal Attainment (King, 1997).

In King's view, the goal of nursing is to assist individuals to attain, maintain, or restore their health. To achieve this outcome, nurses and clients engage in interactions of verbal and nonverbal communication where information is exchanged and interpreted. The outcome of this process is a transaction where values, needs, and wants are shared. King views this interactive process between client and nurse as the essential element of nursing. King (1997) explained the relationship between the four major nursing metaparadigms (humans, nursing, health, and environment) by stating that the domain of nursing involves human beings, families, and communities in a framework where nurses conduct transactions in various environments with the goal of attaining, maintaining, or restoring health.

King wrote that all people grow and develop within nations, which, in turn, make up societies throughout the world, giving a sense of global community. This commonality depicts the communication and interaction that occurs within small groups in their nations' social networks. Three changing and interactive systems, the personal, interpersonal, and social systems, make up most societies throughout the world, according to King (2006).

Assumptions

The assumptions within King's model are many, and for a more complete listing, please refer to King's original sources or Fawcett's chapter on King (Fawcett, 2005; King, 1981, 1997). King's model and Theory of Goal Attainment are based on her overarching belief that the focus of nursing is people interacting with their environment, which leads to a state of health and the ability to function in social roles (King, 1981). A basic assumption of King's Theory of Goal Attainment is that the nurse and client communicate information, set mutual goals, and then act to attain those goals. Factors that affect the attainment of goal are roles, stress, space, and time.

Major assumptions related to the four metaparadigms of nursing are as follows:

Human beings/persons

- Are open, social beings who are unique, rational, sentient, and capable of making decisions

- Have the ability to perceive, think, feel, choose, and set goals and select means to achieve goals
- Have values that are linked to their culture and dictate their behavior and goals
- Differ in their needs, desires, and goals
- Have three fundamental needs, which include the following:
  - Health information
  - Care that seeks to prevent illness
  - Care when they are unable to help themselves

Health

- Is the dynamic life experiences of a human being, which calls for the continuous adjustment to stressors in the internal and external environments causing the optimum use of one's resources to achieve maximum potential for daily living
- Is a changing state where variations are constant and ongoing
- Is made up of genetic, subjective, relative, dynamic, environmental, functional, cultural, and perceptual characteristics (King, 1990)

Environment

- Environment is the background for human interactions.
- Environment involves internal and external components where
  - Internal environment transforms energy to enable humans to adjust to continuous external changes.
  - External environment involves formal and informal organizations and is a source of stress and continuous changes.
- Understanding the ways in which humans interact with their environment to maintain health is necessary for nursing professionals (King, 1981).

Nursing

- Nursing is a goal-seeking system where the performance of roles and responsibilities assists human beings to attain, maintain, and restore health (King, 1971).

- Nursing is a series of actions, reactions, and interactions where the nurse and client exchange information and perceptions and set goals and determine the means to achieve the goals.
- Human beings and their actions are the focus of nursing.

Perceptions of the nurse and the client influence the interaction process (King, 1981, p. 143).

Concepts

King's conceptual model identifies the domain of nursing as a composite of the following three major interacting systems: personal systems (individuals), interpersonal systems (groups), and social systems (society). These three systems provided the basis for King's Theory of Goal Attainment. Humans are the basic element in each of the systems, and the unit of analysis is human behavior in various social environments. King identified 15 concepts and placed them within one of the three systems. However, King readily admits that the concepts are not limited to one system but rather cut across all of the systems.

Personal System

Personal systems are made up of individuals and include the client and nurse functioning as a total system. An individual is described as "a unified being, or self, who perceives, thinks, desires, imagines, decides, and identifies goals to be achieved" (King, 1981, p. 19). A personal system includes seven dimensions, which are perception, self, growth and development, time, body image, learning, and personal space (Fawcett, 2005).

In the personal system, King views the concept of perception as the process of organizing, interpreting, and transforming information from sensory data and memory. Perception is part of the process of human transactions with the environment. Perception gives meaning to one's experience, represents one's image of reality, and influences one's behavior (King, 1981, p. 24). King considered perception to be the most important element within the personal system because of its influence on behavior. One's "perceptions of self, of body image, of time and space influence the way he or she responds to persons, objects, and events in his or her life" (King, 1981, p. 19).

The concept of self is seen as the human being's inner world. Self is who a person perceives himself or herself to be. Growth and development refer to the continuous changes that occur inside and outside of human beings. Growth and development, according to King, include all changes that occur even at the cellular level and are influenced by genetics, lived experiences, and the environment (King, 1981).

Time is the duration between events and is unique to each person. The perception of time is subjective and an irreversible succession of events. Body image is "an individual's perceptions of his/her own body, others' reactions to his/her appearance which results from others' reaction to self" (King, 1981, p. 33). A person's body image is influenced by others' reaction to him or her and the person's interactions with others.

Learning is a "process of sensory perception, conceptualization, and critical thinking involving multiple experiences in which changes in concepts, skills, symbols, habits, and values can be evaluated in observable behaviors and inferred from behavioral manifestations" (King, 1986, p. 24). Personal space is the immediate environment in which nurse and client interact and move toward goal attainment (King, 1981, p. 149). Space exists in all directions, and the physical area or territory communicates role, position, and interactions with others. Space is situational, dimensional, transactional, and dependent on the perception of the person (King, 1981).

Interpersonal System

Interpersonal systems consist of groups or individuals interacting with one another. King (1981) refers to two individuals interacting as dyads, three individuals as triads, and four or more individuals as small or large groups. The more individuals who are involved, the more complex the system becomes.

The concepts associated with interpersonal systems are interaction, transaction, communication, role, coping, and stress. Interactions are the acts of two or more people who are in contact with each other. Interactions occur in concrete situations where human beings are actively participating and moving toward the achievement of a goal. Interactions can reveal how individuals feel about other humans, what expectations exist, and how each reacts to the actions of the other. A transaction is the process of interacting where humans communicate with others and the environment for the purpose of achieving goals that they value. Transactions are goal-directed human behaviors (King, 1981, p. 82). Interactions and transactions between nurse and client constitute an interpersonal system.

Communication is the processing of information where a change occurs from one state to another. According to King (1981), communication is the sharing of thoughts, perceptions, and opinions among individuals using verbal and nonverbal messages to create social interaction and learning opportunities.

Roles are considered a set of behaviors expected from someone who is occupying a certain position in a social framework. Roles are occupied by one or more individuals interacting in a specific setting for a specified purpose. Coping is viewed as a person's ability to handle stressors. Knowledge of coping is necessary for the interpersonal system.

Stress is an energy response of a person to specific people, objects, or events that can be perceived as positive or negative stressors. Stress is a "dynamic state whereby a human being interacts with the environment to maintain balance for growth, development, and performance which involves an exchange of energy and information between the person and the environment for regulation and control of stressors" (King, 1981, p. 98).

Social System

The third interacting system is the social system. Social systems are groups of people within a community or society who share common goals, interests, and values. A social system has organized boundaries, including roles, behaviors, and practices. A social system can be a family, school, or coworkers. The concepts identified within the social systems are organization, authority, power, status, control, and decision making.

An organization can be viewed as a system whose activities are oriented toward the achievement of goals. An organization is made up of a group of human beings with assigned roles and positions who use resources and abilities to accomplish personal and organization goals. Authority is a "transactional process characterized by active, reciprocal relations in which members' values, backgrounds, and perceptions play a role in defining, validating, and accepting the directions of individuals within an organization" (King, 1981, p. 124). Authority is the power to make decisions directing the actions of human beings. Authority may lie in the position one holds or the level of expertise, skill, or depth of knowledge a person possesses.

Power is the ability to use resources to achieve goals. Power is having influence over others in situations. Power defines a situation in a way that people will accept what is being done whether they agree with it or not. Power is situational (King, 1981, p. 127).

Status is the position of a person or a group relative to other groups in an organization. Status is related to who you are, what you do, who you know, and what you have achieved (King, 1981, p. 130). Control is a dimension of the concept of the social system (King, 1986). Decision making is a "dynamic and systematic process by which a goal-directed choice of perceived alternatives is made, and acted upon by individuals or groups to answer a question and attain a goal" (King, 1981, p. 132).

Summary

The relationships between the three systems—personal, interpersonal, and social systems—make up King's Theory of Goal Attainment. The conceptual framework of the interpersonal system had the greatest influence on the development of this theory. King (1981) stated, "Although personal systems and social systems influence quality of care, the major elements in a theory of goal attainment are discovered in the interpersonal systems in which two people, who are usually strangers, come together in a health care organization to help and to be helped to maintain a state of health that permits functioning in roles" (p. 142). King believed that interactions between the nurse and the client led to transactions that resulted in goal attainment and enhanced growth and development of clients.

Nurses have set goals for their patients most likely from the beginning of professional nursing. However, King examined the process of setting goals from a nursing theory perspective and developed a conceptual framework for nursing, out of which arose a usable nursing theory.

King's theory has been used by nurses working in a variety of settings with many different patient populations. While King's theory has been criticized for its vague explanation of environment (Fawcett, 2005) and its inability to be applied to clients who cannot participate in their care (Tomey & Alligood, 2006), nurses have and continue to use King's system and theory to implement theory-based practice.

Theory in Action

Nursing theories are meant to stimulate and support knowledge development related to effectively exploring, predicting, describing, defining, and (sometimes) controlling nursing phenomena. King's work presents an approach to clarifying the process of nurse–patient interaction through collaborative goal identification and planning for attainment. The two historical publications listed below, which are electronically accessible in the major databases, demonstrate King's theory in action:

Temple, A., & Fawdry, M. K. (1992). King's Theory of Goal Attainment: Resolving filial caregiver role strain. *Journal of Gerontological Nursing, 18*(3), 11–15. doi:10.3928/0098-9134-19920301-04

This article applies King's Theory of Goal Attainment to one case involving a geriatric patient and family. Utilization of King's work in this situation helped the involved nurse to clarify role and performance expectations for self, client, and family members.

Alligood, M. R. (2010). Family healthcare with King's Theory of Goal Attainment. *Nursing Science Quarterly, 23*, 99–104. doi:10.1177/0894318410362553

The author describes the application of King's Theory of Goal Attainment in three different family healthcare situations: families with a child with mental illness, a child with type 1 diabetes, and an adult with chronic obstructive pulmonary disease. Productive impact of theory-driven knowledge development is also discussed.

Learning Activities

Locate and read the two articles listed above to see how nurses have used King's work.

1. Recall a client you have cared for recently and briefly list the issues your client had related to each of the dimensions in King's personal system—perception, self, growth and development, time, body image, learning, and personal space.
2. King believed that the interpersonal systems had the greatest influence on a client's quality of care. Do you agree or disagree? Explain your position.
3. Identify the most compelling part of King's Theory of Goal Attainment. Briefly describe the component and explain why you believe this is the most interesting part of King's theory.

References

Fawcett, J. (2005). *Contemporary nursing knowledge: Analysis and evaluation of nursing models and theories* (2nd ed.). Philadelphia, PA: Davis.

King, I. M. (1971). *Toward a theory for nursing: General concepts of human behavior.* Hoboken, NJ: Wiley Publishing.

King, I. M. (1981). *A theory for nursing: Systems, concepts, process.* Hoboken, NJ: J. Wiley Publishing.

King, I. M. (1986). *Curriculum and instruction in nursing: Concepts and processes.* Norwalk, CT: Appleton-Century-Crofts.

King, I. M. (1990). Health as the goal for nursing. *Nursing Science Quarterly,* 3(3), 123–128.

King, I. M. (1997). King's theory of goal attainment in practice. *Nursing Science Quarterly,* 10(4), 180–185.

King, I. M. (2001). The nurse theorists: 21st century updates: Imogene M. King interview by Jacqueline Fawcett. *Nursing Science Quarterly,* 14(4), 311–315.

King, I. M. (2006). A systems approach in nursing administration: Structure, process, and outcome. *Nursing Administration Quarterly,* 30(2), 100–104.

King, I. M. (2007). King's conceptual system, theory of goal attainment and transaction process in the 21st century. *Nursing Science Quarterly,* 20(2), 109–111.

Messmer, P. (2000). Imogene King 1923–2007. In V. L. Bullough & L. Sentz (Eds.), *American nursing: A biographical dictionary* (pp. 164–167). New York, NY: Springer Publishing.

Messmer, P. R. (2009). *Portrait in professionalism: Imogene M. King.* Retrieved from http://www.nursinglibrary.org/vhl/handle/10755/166877

Tomey, A. M., & Alligood, M. R. (2006). *Nursing theorists and their work* (6th ed.). St. Louis, MO: Mosby.

Resources

King International Nursing Group (KING): http://www.kingnursing.org
>   KING was established in the 1990s to foster the development of nursing knowledge based on the work of Dr. Imogene King. It was deactivated for a period of time but was reactivated in August 2009 to honor her work.

Helene Fuld Foundation Portraits of Excellence: Imogene King: Wallace, D. (Producer), & Coberg, T. (Director). (1990). *The nurse theorists: Portraits of excellence* [Motion picture]. United States: Studio Three Productions.
>   Includes King's interview.

Patricia Benner's Model of Skill Acquisition in Nursing

Patricia Sawyer Benner was born in August 1942, in Hampton, Virginia, to Shirley and Clint Sawyer. Her father was a shipbuilder, and she was the middle child with one sister older and one younger than she. Her family moved to Ontario, California, where the Sawyer girls completed their high school education. Her parents divorced when she was a sophomore in high school, which she reported as a very difficult time for all of them. She became interested in becoming a nurse when she worked as an admitting clerk at St. Luke's Hospital while in college. The college she was attending, Pasadena College, did not offer nursing as a major, so she transferred to Pasadena City College, where she obtained her associate of science in nursing degree while simultaneously receiving a bachelor's degree in 1964 from Pasadena College. She went on to earn a master's degree in nursing from the University of California at San Francisco in 1970 and a doctorate at the University of California at Berkeley in 1982.

Benner was one of only a few nurse theorists who married and had children. She married Richard Benner in August 1967, and according to Dr. Benner, her husband's study of situational leadership had a profound effect on her understanding of practice. She has two children, a son born in 1973, and a daughter born in 1981 (Alligood, n.d.).

Benner is currently Professor Emerita at the University of California–San Francisco (UCSF) and has been a nursing professor there since 1982. Benner was the first to hold the Thelma Shobe Endowed Chair in Ethics and Spirituality position at UCSF; she held the position from 2002 until 2008. She is a fellow of the American Academy of Nursing and became an American Nurses Association (ANA) Living Legend in 2011. Since 2004, Benner has served as the director of the Carnegie Foundation's Preparation for the Profession Program. This work focuses on nursing schools' role in the education of nurses. The findings of this research were published in a book entitled *Educating Nurses: A Call for Radical Transformation* in December 2009.

Theoretical Influences

Benner readily acknowledges that her work in model development has been influenced by a number of individuals, including nurse theorist Virginia Henderson and University of California–Berkeley professors Hubert Dreyfus and Stuart Dreyfus, as well as the work of existential philosophers Martin Heidegger, Søren Kierkegaard, and Maurice Merleau-Ponty (Tomey & Alligood, 2006).

Benner studied clinical nursing in an attempt to uncover new knowledge but was very careful to emphasize that practical knowledge without theoretical understanding is problematic. While Benner worked in California, she was introduced to the skill acquisition work of philosopher Hubert Dreyfus and his younger brother, Stuart Dreyfus, an operational engineer. Benner found that skill acquisition is very applicable to nursing. The Dreyfuses' model was developed by studying the processes experts used to play chess as well as armored tank drivers' and airplane pilots' performances in emergency situations.

The Dreyfuses' model is situational and identifies the following five levels of skill acquisition: novice, advanced beginner, competent, proficient, and expert. Movement from one level to the next occurs in several ways. One way is the movement from reliance on abstract principles to the use of past concrete experience as paradigms. The second is a change in the learner's perception of the situation, where the situation is seen less and less as a mass of equally relevant bits and more and more as a complete whole where only certain parts are relevant. The third is a passage from detached observation to involved performer. The performer no longer stands outside the situation but is now engaged in the situation.

Model of Skill Acquisition

Benner adapted the Dreyfuses' model to clinical nursing and in 1984 published her classic book *From Novice to Expert: Excellence and Power in Clinical Nursing Practice*, in which she outlined her model of skill acquisition in nursing. Based on the development of skills outlined by Dreyfus and Dreyfus (1980), Benner was able to describe the process by which nurses learn to practice nursing.

Benner (1984) distinguishes between theoretical knowledge, "knowing that," and practical knowledge, "knowing how," by stating that knowledge development in a practice discipline comes from extending how to do something through scientific investigation based on theory. Benner believes that practical knowledge can extend knowledge and that clinical practice is a rich source for knowledge development. Benner believes that a nurse can be knowledgeable and skillful without ever knowing the theory.

In Benner's model, she identifies seven domains of nursing practice. They are the helping role, teaching-coaching function, diagnostic–patient monitoring function, effective management of rapidly changing situations, administration and monitoring of therapeutic interventions and regimens, monitoring and ensuring the quality of healthcare practices, and organizational and work role competencies (Benner, 1984).

In 1989, Benner extended her model by introducing the concept of caring as a response to stress. Benner worked with Dr. Judith Wrubel on the identification of the existence of caring and its integration into the process of skill acquisition (Benner & Wrubel, 1989).

Skill Acquisition in Nursing

Stage 1: Novice

The first stage of skill acquisition is the novice. In nursing, Benner views novices as beginners, usually students in undergraduate nursing programs, who have no experience with the types of situations in which they are expected to perform. Novices are taught rules to help them perform. The rules are context free and independent of specific cases; hence the rules tend to be rigidly applied in all situations. The rule-governed behavior typical of the novice is extremely limited and inflexible. As such, novices have no life experience in the application of rules. Rules can't tell a novice which tasks to perform in which situations, so behavior in the clinical setting is limited and inflexible, and the novice is oftentimes unable to make the leap from classroom to practice.

Stage 2: Advanced Beginner

Advanced beginners have had enough experiences to discern recurring, meaningful patterns in a situation or to have had them pointed out by a mentor. This usually occurs during the first 6 months after graduation from nursing school. Advanced beginners are beginning to create their own guidelines that can determine their actions. They can perform at a minimal level in real situations. According to Benner (1984), they possess the knowledge, skills, and understanding but lack the in-depth encounters in population.

Stage 3: Competent

After approximately 2–3 years of nursing practice, the competent nurse begins to see the long-term effect of his or her actions in patient situations; however, he or she lacks the efficiency and adaptability seen in proficient nurses. Competent nurses do have a feeling of mastery and can plan and organize effectively. An increasing ability to recognize the salient or most important adds to their effectiveness. They begin to recognize patterns and are able to interpret clinical situations more quickly and accurately.

Stage 4: Proficient

The proficient nurse is able to learn from experiences the expected outcome in a given situation and how one should alter plans in response to events. In the proficient stage of the Dreyfuses' model, nurses view situations in their entirety rather than the component parts. Principles and maxims guide the proficient nurse. The proficient nurse learns from past experiences what events typically occur and how to modify plans in response to different events. The proficient nurse is able to recognize when the expected outcome does not occur. The proficient nurse is able to detect the most important events and subtle nuances and is able to intervene when necessary. This holistic understanding improves the proficient nurse's decision making; however, she must still consciously make decisions. Proficiency usually manifests after 3–4 years of clinical practice.

Stage 5: Expert

The expert performer no longer relies on rules or maxims to make the connection of a situation and needed appropriate intervention. The expert nurse has an intuitive grasp of situations and is able to focus quickly on the correct problem. The expert operates from a deep understanding of the total situation. Experts use rules, guidelines, and maxims only when confronted with a new and unique event. Nurses usually become experts after 5 or more years of clinical practice; however, some nurses never reach expert clinical performance, according to Benner (1984).

Concepts

Benner and Wrubel expanded the model of skill acquisition in nursing by including the concept of caring in nursing practice. Benner and Wrubel defined and described the concepts of caring, nursing, person, health, stress, coping, and situation in a 1989 publication, *The Primacy of Caring: Stress and Coping in Health and Illness,* and used examples of nurse–patient interactions to illustrate the processes and concepts.

Caring

Caring is defined as being connected and having things matter, with fused thoughts, feelings, and action. Caring sets up what is important to a person, and therefore it sets up what is stressful and how a person might cope. Benner and Wrubel (1989) state that all caring rises from connectedness and having some things matter more than others. "Without care, a person would be without projects and concerns. Care . . . sets up meaning distinctions" (Benner & Wrubel, 1989, p. 1).

The behaviors related to caring are characterized by empathy, support, compassion, protection, and nurturance. When a nurse cares for a client, that care creates stress because it is an emotional investment, an engagement process. Engaging with clients makes it possible for nurses to diagnose problems and identify solutions and create a trusting environment. Caring is of primary importance, according to Benner and Wrubel (1989), because it creates the environment where the nurse is able to provide assistance to the client.

Care is primary because it

- Sets up what matters, what is stressful, what options are possible to cope
- Creates an enabling condition of connection and concern
- Sets up the possibility of giving and getting help (Benner & Wrubel, 1989)

Nursing

Nursing is described as a relationship based on caring in an "enabling condition of connection and concern" (Benner & Wrubel, 1989, p. 4). Nursing science is guided by the art and ethics of care and responsibility. "Nurses promote healing through assisting the patient to maintain human ties and concerns and it is the human connection that gives people the courage to weather their illness" (Benner & Wrubel, 1989, p. 87). The relationship of health, illness, and disease is central to Benner and Wrubel's view of nursing practice.

Person

Benner and Wrubel's interpretation of *person* is based on existential philosophy and the oneness or wholeness of human beings. Benner thus describes person as "a self-interpreting being, that is, the person does not come into the world predefined but gets defined in the course of living a life" (Benner & Wrubel, 1989, p. 41). A person is viewed as a creative, generative being who lives in the context of meaning and whose actions and understandings form a comprehensible whole. Benner and Wrubel (1989) characterize the person as someone who must deal with situations, body, personal concerns, and the temporary nature of events.

Health

Benner and Wrubel (1989) use Kleinman, Eisenberg, and Good's definition of health as "health [is] not the absence of illness and illness is not identical with disease" (p. 8). Illness is described as the experience of loss or dysfunction, whereas disease is the manifestation of aberration at the cellular, tissue, or organ level. All treatment for disease and illness must make sense within the context of the lived human experience.

Situation

Benner uses situation, rather than the concept of environment, in her work. Benner chose situation because, according to Benner, situation has a social context with meaning and interpretation, which affects people. People "inhabit their world, rather than live in an environment" (Benner & Wrubel, 1989, p. 49). A person's interpretation influences each situation. Benner's phenomenologically based view of situation is evident in her writing when she uses the terms *being situated* and *situated meaning*, indicating a person's engagement with and interpretation of each life event.

Stress

According to Benner and Wrubel (1989), stress is "the disruption of meanings, understanding, and smooth functioning so that harm, loss, or challenge is experienced, and sorrow, interpretation, or new skill acquisition is required" (p. 59). Stress is viewed as the physical, emotional, and/or intellectual realization that smooth functioning has been disrupted. Stress occurs when the person understands that something is amiss or out of balance. Stress is the inevitable consequence of living in a world where one cares about things, and therefore it cannot be eliminated.

Coping

Coping is not considered an antidote for stress but rather what one does about the disruption caused by the stress. Benner and Wrubel draw on the work of Lazarus (1966) to explain stress and coping. Coping is "doing something directly" as well as "not doing something on purpose" (Benner & Wrubel, 1989, p. 62). Other coping behaviors are seeking information, reframing the way one views the situation, and making a choice to have a positive attitude in the face of the disruption. Benner and Wrubel (1989) give numerous examples of how one copes with various situations such as development across the life span, caregiving itself, various symptoms, cancer, and neurologic illnesses, among others.

Summary

Benner's work on skill acquisition and stress, coping, and caring offers insight into these complex and important issues derived directly from nursing practice. Although some have criticized Benner's work of the "intuitive knower" as leading to subjective understanding of nursing knowledge without empirical validation and her form of phenomenologic understanding of nursing practice, the Benner model can help nurses understand how expertise develops, allowing them to support and nurture each other (Reed & Shearer, 2009). Benner's work on skill acquisition has been extremely helpful to nurse educators and administrators in knowing more about how students and nurses learn and advance in their knowledge over their careers, and her work with Wrubel on caring represents a totally new view of this central concept.

Benner's model has led to the development of nursing competencies in multiple domains and has expanded to reflect advanced practice and critical care nursing (Benner, 1984; Benner, Hooper-Kyriakidis, & Stannard, 1999; Brykczynski, 1999). Benner's work also validated the value of narrative accounts of nursing in expanding nursing knowledge and the central role of caring in the practice of nursing.

Theory in Action

Nursing theories are meant to stimulate and support knowledge development related to effectively exploring, predicting, describing, defining, and (sometimes) controlling nursing phenomena. Benner's work clarifies stages of professional development in nursing and has provided needed structure for knowledge development related to better understanding how nurses learn to become excellent at what they do. The two publications listed below, which are electronically accessible in the major databases, demonstrate Benner's theory in action:

Larrabee, S. B. (1999). Benner's novice to expert nursing theory applied to implementation of laptops in the home care setting. *Home Health Care Management Practice*, 11, 41–47. doi:10.1177/108482239901100510

This historical article applies Benner's model to the process of nurses in home healthcare learning to use laptop computers to record patient information during a time when laptops were just being introduced as a way to record patient data in the field instead of using written notes. Novice to expert guidelines are presented to explore and establish guidelines for nurses, staff, and administration.

Carlson, L., Crawford, N., & Contrades, S. (1989). Nursing student novice to expert: Benner's research applied to education. *Journal of Nursing Education*, 28(4), 188–190.

During the process of nursing education, students are sometimes too overwhelmed to see their own knowledge and skill development. In this article, Benner's Novice to Expert Model is presented as a paradigm that helps educators and students envision clinical practice as a developmental process and become better aware of educational progress.

Learning Activities

Locate and read the two articles listed above to see how nurses have used Benner's work.

1. Think of the first time you were to give a hospitalized patient an oral medication. Recall your preparation and comfort related to that task. Now compare that experience to giving a patient an oral medication today. Discuss the growth you have experienced in your skill level.
2. Recall nurses you have seen caring for different patients. Give examples of situations where a nurse noticed a subtle change in a patient's condition that you had overlooked and reflect on what clues the nurse must have noticed that you did not pick up on.

3. One of Benner's assumptions is that all caring rises from connectedness and having some things matter more than others. Do you agree or disagree, and why?

References

Alligood, M. R. (Interviewer). (nd). *The nurse theorists: Portrait of excellence* (Vol. 2). Interview with Patricia Benner. Helene Fuld Foundation FITNE.

Benner, P. (1984). *From novice to expert: Excellence and power in clinical nursing practice.* Menlo Park, CA: Addison-Wesley.

Benner, P., Hooper-Kyriakidis, P., & Stannard, D. (1999). *Clinical wisdom in critical care: A thinking-in-action approach.* Philadelphia, PA: W. B. Saunders.

Benner, P., & Wrubel, J. (1989). *The primacy of caring: Stress and coping in health and illness.* Menlo Park, CA: Addison-Wesley.

Brykczynski, L. A. (1999). An interpretive study describing the clinical judgment of nursing practitioners. *Scholarly Inquiry for Nursing Practice: An International Journal,* 13(2), 141–166.

Dreyfus, S. E., & Dreyfus, H. I. (1980). *A five-stage model of the mental activities involved in directed skill acquisition.* Unpublished report. Berkeley: University of California at Berkeley.

Lazaras, R. S. (1966). *Psychological stress and the coping process.* New York, NY: McGraw-Hill.

Reed, P. G. & Shearer, N. B. C. (2009). *Perspectives on Nursing Theory* (5th ed.). Philadelphia, PA: Lippincott, Williams, and Wilkins.

Tomey, A. M., & Alligood, M. R. (2006). *Nursing theorists and their work* (6th ed.). St. Louis, MO: Mosby.

Web Resources

Benner Associates consulting firm: http://home.earthlink.net/~bennerassoc/

Hubert Dreyfus homepage: http://socrates.berkeley.edu/~hdreyfus/

Dr. Dreyfus was awarded Dickson Emeriti Professorship, 2009–2010, University of California–Berkley.

Patricia Benner's faculty profile: http://nursing.ucsf.edu/news/american-academy-nursing-designates-dr-patricia-benner-living-legend

CHAPTER

23

Afaf Ibrahim Meleis's Transitions Theory

Afaf Ibrahim Meleis was born on March 19, 1942, in Alexandria, Egypt (Masters, 2015). Both of Meleis's parents were accomplished individuals. Her father began his professional career as a director of lighthouses and served in the Egyptian Navy on a ship called the Aida. He rose to the rank of director general. Her father was "very handsome" and popular with the ladies (Afaf Ibrahim Meleis, personal communication, May 1, 2015). He was able to put his naval career on hold and care for Meleis and her sister when they were 12 and 3 years old, respectively, so that the girls' mother could attend Syracuse University in New York to get the first Bachelor of Science degree in nursing ever awarded to a nurse from the Middle East. This shaped Meleis's commitment to a professional career (Afaf Ibrahim Meleis, personal communication, May 1, 2015). Meleis was heavily influenced by her mother, who went on to become the first Egyptian nurse to earn a Master of Public Health degree and doctorate from an Egyptian university (Im, 2014). Meleis also has an accomplished sister, who is happily married and living in San Diego, California. Her sister is a sociologist who conducts hospital-based sociological research and guides historical tours to Egypt using her expertise as an Egyptologist (Afaf Ibrahim Meleis, personal communication, May 1, 2015).

Like other nursing theorists and leaders, Meleis's parents were not pleased with her choice to become a nurse, but she was not dissuaded.

Meleis graduated magna cum laude from the University of Alexandria in 1961 (Im, 2014). She left Egypt in the early 1960s to pursue graduate education in nursing at the University of California, Los Angeles. She earned a Master of Science degree in nursing in 1964, a Master of Arts degree in sociology in 1966, and a doctorate in medical and social psychology in 1968 from the University of California, Los Angeles (Meleis, 2010).

Meleis served as a faculty member at the University California, Los Angeles, from 1966 to 1971, and in 1971, she moved to the University of California, San Francisco, where she taught for the next 34 years. During this time she developed her Transitions Theory. Meleis served as the fifth dean of the top-ranked University of Pennsylvania School of Nursing from 2002 until 2014, when she stepped out of that role and is currently serving as Professor of Nursing and Sociology at the University of Pennsylvania (University of Pennsylvania School of Nursing, 2008).

Meleis has been married for more than 50 years to a nuclear engineer, Dr. Mahmoud Meleis, and they have two sons and grandchildren (Meleis, 2012). Her husband has been supportive throughout her career and continues to encourage her daily (Afaf Ibrahim Meleis, personal communication, May 1, 2015).

Her scholarship has been focused in several areas, including women's health, international health, and theoretical development of nursing. She has authored more than 175 articles published in social science, nursing, and medical journals and has written more than 40 chapters and 7 books. Meleis has mentored hundreds of students, clinicians, and researchers from the United States, Thailand, Brazil, Egypt, Jordan, Israel, Colombia, South Korea, and Japan (University of Pennsylvania School of Nursing, 2008).

Meleis is a fellow in the American Academy of Nursing and in 1990 received the Medal of Excellence for professional and scholarly achievements from Egyptian President Hosni Mubarak. She received the 2008 Commission on Graduates of Foreign Nursing Schools International Distinguished Leadership Award based on her outstanding work in the global healthcare community. In 2010, she was inducted into the UCLA School of Nursing Hall of Fame for her work in advancing and transforming nursing science (Im, 2014).

Professor and creator of the Behavioral System Model Dorothy Johnson asked Meleis to take over the teaching of her "one-of-a-kind" Nursing

Theory class in the School of Nursing at UCLA in 1966, just 1 year after Meleis had finished her doctorate. It was the experience of teaching nursing theory that ignited Meleis's passion for nursing theory and passing knowledge of nursing theory on to students (Afaf Ibrahim Meleis, personal communication, May 1, 2015).

Dr. Ralph H. Turner, a UCLA sociologist and one of the founders of the collective behavior and social movement, served as Meleis's "theoretical guru" and was the person who inspired her interest in role and theory development (Meleis, 2010; UCLA Newsroom, 2014). Turner also became and remained a very close friend until his death in his 90s (Afaf Ibrahim Meleis, personal communication, May 1, 2015).

Meleis attributes her passion for theory-based research to a mentor and another dear family friend, psychologist Burton Meyer. Dr. Meyer was hired by the then Dean of Nursing at UCLA, Dr. Lula Wolf Hassenplug, to teach research. Meyer taught the need for a conceptual framework in research, which was a new idea in the 1960s. Meleis's association with Meyer was relatively short-lived, however. Meyer died suddenly in 1967 of pancreatic cancer after knowing Meleis for only 5 short years. But his influence as her mentor left an indelible mark on her career (Afaf Ibrahim Meleis, personal communication, May 1, 2015, and May 13, 2015).

Transitions Theory

Meleis began developing her view of Transitions Theory during her doctoral studies at UCLA in the mid-1960s. As she worked as a nurse and researcher, she interviewed women around the globe. She paid particular attention to the transitions in their situations and life experiences, their responses to those transitions, and how those transitions related to their health. This led her to become an advocate and specialist in women's health and to begin crafting the basis of what would become Transitions Theory.

Nurses everywhere generously provided her with their stories about patients' admissions, discharges, plans of care, and so forth. Those stories inspired her to develop Transitions Theory (Afaf Ibrahim Meleis, personal communication, May 1, 2015).

The development of Transitions Theory was guided by three patterns of thought: role theory, lived experiences, and feminist postcolonialism.

1. Role theory incorporates how clients transition from one role to another.
2. Lived experiences focus on the responses to change and the experiences of the people going through the change.
3. Feminist postcolonialism is about power relationships, oppression, and discrimination and how those issues relate to race, ethnicity, nationality, and gender (Meleis, 2015, pp. 362–363).

Basic Beliefs

Transitions Theory is a mid-range theory that has been well received by nurse researchers and used as the conceptual basis in many research articles (Im, 2014). The concept of transitions is central to the practice of nursing (Meleis, 2012). Transitions Theory proposes that certain events trigger transitions. This movement is generally viewed as positive because completion of transitions results in greater stability (Meleis, 2010). Transitions that relate to health, self-care, or well-being may result in interactions with nurses.

Definitions

Transitions Theory offers a framework in which to organize the experiences of individuals, families, groups, organizations, and communities that are facing and coping with events, situations, or developmental milestones that require new skills, knowledge, or ways of thinking or being (Meleis, 2015). *Transition* is defined as "a passage from one life phase, condition, or status to another, a multiple concept embracing the elements of process, time span and perception" (Chick & Meleis, 1986, p. 25). There are four different types of transitions: developmental, situational, health–illness, and organizational transitions. Developmental transitions occur as a normal part of growing and developing as individuals progress through the stages of life. Developmental transitions include adolescence, adulthood, and becoming a father, for example. Situational transitions are triggered by an event that has health–illness implications, such as a heart attack or hometown being hit by a tornado. Organizational transitions are ones in which the environment or groups are affected by rules and regulations governing them in some way. For example, getting a new supervisor or implementing new policies at work.

Assumptions

Transitions Theory has 11 assumptions:

1. A client's response to various transitions is shaped by interactions with others and reference groups.
2. Change, through health–illness events and situations, triggers a process before and after the event itself.
3. Individuals and/or families experience a change process with different responses and outcomes even if they are not aware of the triggering event or response.
4. The nature of the experience shapes the outcome.
5. Prevention actions and therapeutic interventions can affect outcomes.
6. Clients have the capacity to assume new roles as shaped by their environment.
7. Health care can be delivered more equitably by using well-documented evidence.
8. Gender, race, culture, heritage, and sexual orientation shape people's experiences with the healthcare system and therefore their health outcome.
9. Humanism, holism, context, health, well-being, goals, and care are all part of nursing's purview.
10. Environment is defined as the physical, social, cultural, organizational, and societal factors that influence experiences, interventions, and outcomes.
11. Recipients of nursing care are individuals, families, and communities, and they are partners in the care processes (Meleis, 2015, p. 363).

Properties/Concepts

Although the types of transitions are different, they have similarities. These similarities are called properties and have been supported in the literature (Schumacher & Meleis, 1994). Meleis identifies these properties as concepts in her most recent work on the theory (Meleis, 2015). The five properties/concepts are *time span*, or that transitions develop over time, and that transitions are *fluid processes*, flowing from one state to another, having stages. There is also a *feeling of disconnectedness* that may be real or perceived isolation. The fourth property is *awareness*, where individuals and/or families are aware that they are experiencing the triggering event, situation, or change and what is or has happened to them. The fifth property is *presence of milestones* that could serve as a place where the individual, family, or organization could begin to turn things around. Knowing appropriate milestones is essential to helping people move through transitions successfully (Meleis, 2015).

The literature also indicates that individuals' and families' identities, roles relationships, abilities, and patterns of behavior change during transitions (Schumacher & Meleis, 1994). As a response to transitions, organizations change the way they are organized, internal or external relationships, and the way they operate.

Definitions related to the four metaparadigms of nursing are described in the following subsections.

Nursing

Nursing is a human science that focuses on health-related life experiences, their meanings, and their significance, including the experience of dying. Nurses are concerned with how these experiences shape the actions and reactions of individuals. This concern makes nursing practice a discipline and helps to define its perspective (Meleis, 2012). Nursing's goal is that the "client emerge from any nursing encounter not only more comfortable and better able to deal with the present health problem, but also better equipped to protect and promote health for the future" (Chick & Meleis, 1986, p. 31).

Person

Meleis does not explicitly define person in her work but she does speak about the client of nursing. A nursing client is defined as a human being who has needs, is in constant interaction with the environment and with the ability to adapt to those surroundings but is due to illness, risk or vulnerability from illness, actual or potential, is experiencing or is at risk for disequilibrium (Meleis, 2012).

Health

In Meleis's keynote address at the Discovery International Nurse Theorist Conference in May 1989, she proposed the need for multiple definitions of health based on the clinical setting, culture, and patient environment and further stated that a "quest for a single definition of health is not appropriate, possible, or useful" (Meleis, 1990, p. 109). Meleis views health as a continuum, the central goal of nursing, and more than the absence of disease (Chick & Meleis, 1986; Meleis, 2012). Health results in personal empowerment and a sense of well-being according to Meleis (Afaf Ibrahim Meleis, personal email communication, June 3, 2015). Any definition of health must encompass an understanding of those who are underrepresented and underserved, the role lack of resources plays on well-being, women's rights, and the dynamic nature of life (Meleis, 1990).

Environment

At stated in the list of assumptions, environment is viewed as "the physical, social, cultural, organizational, and societal factors that influence experiences, interventions, and outcomes" (Meleis, 2015, p. 363). One is also able to infer from Meleis's writings that environments are not static and are constantly changing. Chick and Meleis (1986) specifically link transitions to the environment in two ways. First, the environment can cause, or contribute to, a transition, such as a flood or limb falling, resulting in a person becoming a paraplegic. The speed of the change, whether fast or slow, may prompt the transition, with rapid changes usually requiring a greater adjustment. Second, the change inherent within the transition may change what the environment offers in terms of support. For example, in the case of a flood, people may lose access to normal support systems if they must live in a shelter while displaced.

Responses to Transitions

There are two types of responses to transitions: process patterns and outcome patterns. Process patterns are measured by the extent of engagement in the change event, level of confidence in handling situations, and new demands. Process patterns occur during the transition, and outcome patterns are assessed at the end of the transition process.

Mastery, fluid integrative identities, resourcefulness, healthy interactions, and perceived well-being are patterns of outcome responses (Meleis, Sawyer, Im, Schumacher, & Messias, 2000). Assessing process indicators is important because it can alert the nurse to whether the client is moving toward risk, illness, and unhealthy outcomes or toward health, perceived well-being, and healthy outcomes.

Interventions

Healthy outcomes during transitions is the goal. To facilitate this, interventions may be necessary. Clarifying roles, goal setting, providing expertise, role modeling, providing resources, accessing reference groups, debriefing, and rehearsing are all suggested nursing interventions to be used during transitions. Transition Theory uses critical points or milestones throughout the care pathway where special attention, education, intervention, or evaluation is necessary to prevent a reversal of progress (Meleis, 2015). Examples of milestones are newborn checkup or 6 weeks recovery for heart attack. Debriefing is an interviewing method whereby people are allowed to talk about the circumstances surrounding a critical encounter repeatedly as needed. Debriefing is very helpful during a transition at milestones to facilitate emotional well-being (Meleis, 2010). Sharing one's stressful experiences is very important in helping people accept the reality of the situation, express their feelings, and gain perspective on issues.

Clinical Applications

There are many clinical applications of Transition Theory. It has been applied effectively to the care of individuals, families, groups, communities, and organizations experiencing transitions. Transitions Theory assists health professionals to view the client situation from a wholistic perspective, considering the caregiver's beliefs, experiences, points of views, and desired outcomes. Through the Transitions lens, nurses and others can allocate resources and plan care designed specifically to meet caregivers' specific needs so that the health of the patient and the caregiver are enhanced (Blum & Sherman, 2010). An example of a person going through a significant transition is a patient scheduled to have a colectomy. The patient most likely will be aware of his transition but perhaps not the scope of the upcoming change. The nurse can arrange for an enterostomal therapist, if available, to consult with the patient. The patient's changes and differences are examined when the nurse encourages him to speak about his feelings related to the surgery. The patient may perceive himself to be different and not "whole." There will be a period of presurgery, inpatient status, recovery, and adjustment that will be managed by different personnel. The patient will need different therapeutics at each level specific to his care at that time. Critical points and events are when the patient has become accustomed and adapted to his new way of life. The period of transition will be marked by the alteration in body function and in the process of healing, recovery, and learning new ways of coping.

Nursing Education

Schools of nursing have used Transitions Theory as the conceptual framework upon which to base their program of studies. The theory and its components are clear, and nursing courses can easily be arranged using the concepts within the Transitions framework. Many doctoral students, including students in other countries such as Sweden, choose Transitions Theory as the theoretical basis for their doctoral dissertations (Meleis, 2015). The University of Connecticut in Storrs is currently using Transitions Theory (Meleis, 2015), and the University of Massachusetts Boston Undergraduate Nursing program faculty proposed a curricular redesign in 2015 and is planning to adopt a concept-based curriculum change based on Meleis's Transitions framework in the near future (Jacqueline Fawcett, personal communication, April 30, 2015).

Clayton State University School of Nursing, in Atlanta, Georgia, has used Meleis's Transitions Theory as the basis for its curriculum for more than 15 years. The theory serves as the conceptual framework for both its graduate and undergraduate programs. The faculty in the undergraduate program have chosen to design all of the major clinical nursing courses around types of transitions, entitling the courses Health–Illness Transitions I, II, and III, Developmental Transitions I and II, Organizational Transitions, Psycho-Social Transitions, and Role Transitions. This curricular model has been extremely successful with consistently positive outcomes and very high National Council Licensure Examination (NCLEX) pass rates.

The University of Pennsylvania established the New Courtland Center for Transitions and Health in 2007 from a $5 million endowment, with research being targeted toward patients with chronic illnesses (Im, 2014). The center states by "using multiple research methods, the research members are creating a body of knowledge using Transitions Theory that will directly benefit patients" (University of Pennsylvania School of Nursing, 2008).

Summary

Meleis's Transitions Theory is a mid-range nursing theory that is popular because of its ease of use, simplicity, and wide applicability to a variety of patients across cultures. The methodologies are clear, concise, and not terribly abstract. Transitions Theory, developed through induction, looks at the passages in life caused by change, growth and development, situations, illness, and disruption in organizations that affect lives. Meleis's theory offers a very useful way of organizing the events that affect all people, causing disequilibrium and movement toward illness. Unhealthy outcomes can be avoided if nurses can assist patients in adapting to their transitions. No doubt as more and more nurses use the theory in practice and research, Transitions Theory will continue to offer a very practical perspective for nurses to consider.

Theory in Action

Nursing theories are meant to stimulate and support knowledge development related to effectively exploring, predicting, describing, defining, and (sometimes) controlling nursing phenomena. Transitions Theory has served as a theoretical framework extensively. Two recent and interesting research studies are as follows:

Ramsey, P., Huby, G., Thompson, A., & Walsh, T. (2014). Intensive care survivors' experiences of ward-based care: Meleis' theory of nursing transitions and role development among critical care outreach services. *Journal of Clinical Nursing*, 23(5–6), 605–615. doi:10.1111/jocn.12452

This article focuses on the psychosocial needs of discharged ICU patients receiving outreach, follow-up debriefing.

Rose, K. M., & Lopez, R. P. (2012). Transitions in dementia care: Theoretical support for nursing roles. *Online Journal in Nursing*, 17(2). doi:10.3912/OJIN .Vol17No02Man04

In this article, the concept of transitional care and how it relates to nursing care of older adults with Alzheimer's disease and other dementias is explored. A brief description of Transitions Theory with a dementia trajectory is given along with evidence for expanding nursing roles in transitions and recommendations for further research.

Learning Activities

Locate and read the two articles listed above to see how nurses have used Meleis's work.

1. Choose one of Meleis's types of transitions and give an example of one such transition. Be prepared to defend your answer.
2. Select a medical condition or transition with which you are familiar and identify the appropriate milestones or critical points a nurse would expect to see in the normal course of that disease or transition.
3. Discuss one idea or concept expressed by Meleis that caused you to think more deeply about a client situation you might have encountered. How might your approach to your patient or client have been different if viewed through Transitions Theory?

References

Blum, K., & Sherman, D. (2010). Understanding the experience of caregivers: A focus on transitions. *Seminars in Oncology Nursing*, 26(4), 243–258.

Chick, N., & Meleis, A. I. (1986). Transitions: A nursing concern. In P. L. Chinn (ed.), *Nursing research methodology* (pp. 237–257). Boulder, CO: Aspen.

Im, E. O. (2014). Afaf Ibrahim Meleis: Transition theory. In M. R. Alligood (Ed.), *Nursing theorists and their work* (8th ed., pp. 378–395). Maryland Heights, MO: Mosby.

Masters, K. (2015). *Nursing theories: A framework for professional practice* (2nd ed.). Burlington, MA: Jones & Bartlett Learning.

Meleis, A. I. (1990). Being and becoming healthy: The core of nursing knowledge. *Nursing Science Quarterly*, 3(3), 107–114.

Meleis, A. I. (2010). *Transitions theory: Middle-range and situation-specific theories in nursing research and practice*. New York, NY: Springer.

Meleis, A. I. (2012). *Theoretical nursing: Development and process* (5th ed.). Philadelphia, PA: Lippincott Williams & Wilkins.

Meleis, A. I. (2015). In M. C. Smith & M. E. Parker (Eds.), *Nursing theories and nursing practice* (4th ed., pp. 362–363). Philadelphia, PA: F. A. Davis.

Meleis, A. I., Sawyer, L., Im, E., Schumacher, K., & Messias, D. (2000). Experiencing transitions: An emerging middle-range theory. *Advances in Nursing Science*, 23(1), 12–28.

Schumacher, K. L., & Meleis, A. I. (1994). Transitions: A central concept of nursing. *Image: Journal of Nursing Scholarship*, 26(2), 119–127.

UCLA Newsroom. (2014, November 19). In memoriam: UCLA sociologist Ralph Turner. Retrieved from http://newsroom.ucla.edu/stories/in-memoriam-ucla-sociologist-ralph-turner

University of Pennsylvania School of Nursing. (2008). *New Courtland Center for Transitions and Health*. Philadelphia, PA: Author.

Theories That Defy Classification

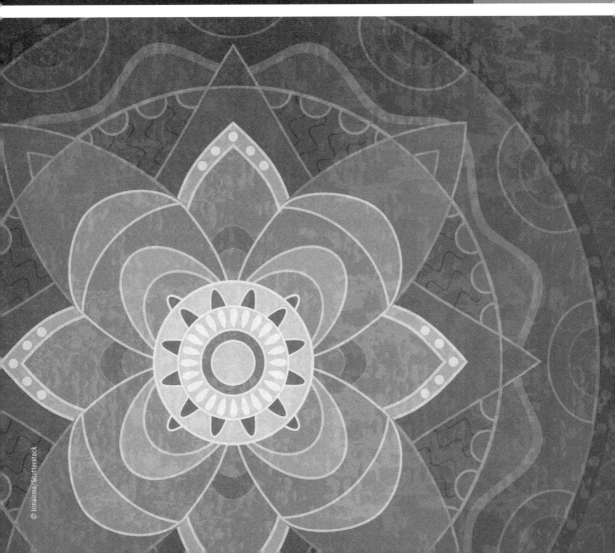

Envisioning Theories That Defy Classification Through Space Photography

"Theories that defy classification" is not a phrase traditionally used to describe nursing theories. Martha Rogers's Unitary Human Beings and Margaret Newman's Health as Expanding Consciousness are discussed in this section of the text because they are both unusually progressive and groundbreaking. The concepts proposed in these theories broadly encompass facets of philosophy, theoretical physics, spirituality, health/wellness, wholism, nondualism, and alternative approaches to understanding the universe. Because of the ongoing theoretical exploration and boundary testing associated with these theories, it is not possible to place them in any of the three traditional classifications previously discussed. These same attributes have made them somewhat difficult to understand, controversial, and not directly applicable to practice.

However, these theories are valuable to the nursing profession because they challenge traditional thinking, spawn professional debate, and provide fresh possibilities for future conceptualizations of nursing.

Envision space photography when exploring nursing theories that defy classification. When trying to understand such theories, one can envision space photography, noting its nebulous, undefined nature. Photos of the cosmos taken with telescopes convey boundlessness and the notion of a new frontier, much like Rogers's and Newman's theories. The Hubble Space Telescope has taken thousands of stunning photographs of space, reaching into the far corners of the universe (see **Color Plates 23** and **24** in the color insert).

No matter from how far away the images come, there is still more beyond to reach out to—the unending darkness and glowing shapes just out of focusing range of the camera. Theories that defy classification are much the same; they propose new, limitless perceptions of nursing and humanity and have philosophical boundaries that are blurry and ever expanding.

Perform a Web search using the phrase *Hubble Space Telescope*. Visit one of a number of sites with Hubble Space Telescope galleries that offer photographs for viewing. Envision these photographs as visual representations of progressive theories that challenge the traditional boundaries of accepted thinking and reasoning in nursing and health care.

When exploring theories that defy classification, ask these questions:

1. What aspects of humanity are explored in the theory?
2. What are the central concepts that form the basis of the theory?
3. Is there an overall theme that governs perceptions of the central concepts?
4. How might the propositions expressed in this theory affect everyday nursing practice?
5. Does the theory resonate with your own experience?

Learning Activities

1. Perform an Internet search using the phrase *Hubble Space Telescope* to find stunning photographs of outer space taken from the Hubble Space Telescope. Print four of your favorite photos.

Martha Rogers's Unitary Human Beings

M artha Rogers (1914–1994) was born in Dallas, Texas. She received her diploma in nursing from Knoxville, Tennessee, General Hospital School of Nursing in 1936. She earned her Bachelor of Science degree in nursing from George Peabody College in Nashville, Tennessee, in 1937. Rogers earned a Master of Arts degree in public health nursing supervision in 1954 from Teachers College, Columbia University, New York. She then earned a master's degree in public health (MPH) in 1952 and Doctor of Science degree in 1954 from Johns Hopkins University in Baltimore. Rogers's early nursing practice was in the area of rural community health nursing. From 1954 to 1975, she was professor and head of the division of nursing at New York University. After 1975, Rogers was a professor at New York University, becoming Professor Emerita in 1979. She held this title until her death at the age of 79 (Tomey & Alligood, 2002). Over her long career, Rogers published more than 200 articles and 3 books. She also received many awards for her contributions to nursing.

Rogers was a nurse visionary who created an innovative conceptual system that continues to influence the nursing profession today. Rogers's model is supported by continued development of similar ideas associated with chaos theory and quantum physics. Rogers loved the color purple and dreamed of nursing in space. She created an innovative conceptual system that views humans as energy fields identified by patterns.

The first question in discussing Rogers's Unitary Human Beings might be: What does the word *unitary* mean? Rogers used the word *unitary* to describe human beings as intrinsically whole rather than a sum of parts. Information about physiologic functioning or a person's social background may be helpful in providing care; however, this information does not impart full understanding of the unitary human being. To understand Rogers's concepts, it becomes necessary to shift one's perception from viewing a client as the sum of many parts to viewing the client and his or her environment as infinite energy fields with no physical boundaries.

Nine assertions about the nature of humankind and human life form the basis of Unitary Human Beings (Biley, 2002; Tomey & Alligood, 2002):

1. *Wholeness* refers to when a person is thought of as being different and more than a sum of parts.
2. *Openness* describes the continual interchange of matter and energy between the individual and the environment.
3. *Unidirectionality* describes the assertion that the life process is not reversible, similar to a car driving down a one-way street that cannot back up.
4. *Pattern and organization* identifies individuals and reflects fluid, ever-changing wholeness.
5. *Sentience and thought* is a human trait—human beings being the only living creatures capable of imagination, abstraction, language, thought, sensation, and emotion.
6. *One energy field* that is infinite constitutes all matter, both living and nonliving. There are two kinds of fields: the human field and the environmental field.
7. *Universe of open systems* describes infinite groups of energy fields that interact with one another continuously.
8. *Patterns* define unique energy fields. Patterns change continuously, giving identity to human environmental energy fields.
9. *The pandimension* is an infinite domain and contains all energy fields. It fully represents the unitary whole.

Basic definitions of three key terms may be helpful in clarifying specific concepts (Biley, 2002):

- A *person* is more than a sum of parts, and it is impossible to divide a person into parts and still be able to understand the whole person.

- The *environment* is a wave pattern. The pattern changes continuously. Each human field pattern is unique and is seamlessly intertwined with its own unique environmental field pattern.
- *Nursing* is an organized body of abstract knowledge, used for the purpose of "assisting human beings to move in the direction of maximum well-being" (Rogers, 1994, p. 64).

Rogers did not specifically mention the notions of *health, wellness,* or *illness* in her writings. Many scholars believe that this is because levels of illness and wellness are based on social definitions and probably encourage the tendency to view a person as a "sum of parts" rather than as a unitary being.

Nursing actions based on Rogers's Unitary Human Beings include the following (Cowling, 1990):

1. Interventions that arise from the nurse's awareness of continuously interacting energy fields based on patterns rather than age, disease process, gender, or other factors
2. Awareness of the influence of individual perceptions, experiences, and modes of expression
3. Actions based on all modes of sentient awareness, including the five senses and intuition, feelings, thoughts, imagination, memories, and any other expressions of human awareness
4. Pattern recognition involving all human ways of knowing that is continuous and based in reality
5. Assessments communicated verbally or through visual input
6. Assessments created by the nurse that are either accepted or not accepted by the client
7. Interventions based on mutual nurse and client acceptance of assessments
8. Ongoing evaluation and reevaluation of assessments and actions with continual input from self, environment, and client

In summary, Rogers's innovative approach to understanding humanity, and nursing's place in it, has illuminated new horizons of inquiry within all nursing practice settings (George, 2002). Within the framework of Rogers's Unitary Human Beings, the function of nursing becomes that of recognizing patterns of energy within client and self and then mutually acting to guide and redirect these patterns to support optimum functioning. Rogers broadened the concept of wholism in nursing by essentially removing the notion that a "whole" entity must be composed of a grouping of parts and asserting that all things are intrinsically whole and seamlessly connected with all that is. In 1966, Rogers wrote the following about nursing:

> Nursing's story is a magnificent epic of service to mankind. It is about people: How they are born, and live, and die; in health and in sickness; in joy and in sorrow. Its mission is the translation of knowledge into human service.
>
> Nursing is compassionate concern for human beings. It is the heart that understands and the hand that soothes. It is the intellect that synthesizes many learnings into meaningful ministrations.*

Here is one way to visualize a Rogerian universe: envision outer space, a black limitless background without boundary. Orbs of light appear at various depths. Some of the orbs are bright white, others a cool blue or green, and still others are yellow, red, and orange. Superimpose over this entire universe a finely woven, four-dimensional matrix made of extremely fine silver thread. Each of the orbs in this universe exists in, around, and through the netting. Envision the net and all it contains flexing, undulating, and becoming alternately dense and thin in an unending dance of interaction and movement. None of what makes up this universe disappears, and no new entities appear. There is just gentle shifting of movement and the gradual, irreversible transformation of orbs and netting in a continual journey of manifest completeness.

Theory in Action

Nursing theories are meant to stimulate and support knowledge development related to effectively exploring, predicting, describing, defining, and (sometimes) controlling nursing phenomena. Rogers envisioned a vast world of energetic interplay and then related it to nursing in ways that could be understood and applied in everyday practice. The two historic publications listed below, which are electronically accessible in the major databases, demonstrate Rogers's theory in action:

Yarcheski, A., Mahon, N. E., & Yarcheski, T. J. (2004). Health and well-being in early adolescents using Rogers' Science of Unitary Beings. *Nursing Science Quarterly*, 17, 72–77. doi:10.1177/0894318403260473

---

*Rogers, M. E. (1966). Doctoral education in nursing. *Nursing Forum*, 5(2), 75–82. Reprinted by permission of John Wiley and Sons.

This article presents a study in which early adolescent participants provided information related to perceived health status, health conception, and well-being. Results validated the evolving concept that the term *well-being* is more compatible in Rogers's theoretical construct than is the term *health*.

Willis, D. G., & Griffith, C. A. (2010). Healing patterns revealed in middle school boys' experiences of being bullied using Rogers' Science of Unitary Human Beings. *Journal of Child and Adolescent Psychiatric Nursing*, 23(3), 125–132. doi:10.1111/j.1744-6171.2010.00234.x

A phenomenological study approach was utilized to collect and analyze evidence related to bullying and healing in middle school boys. Identified patterns of healing included meaning making, self-transcendence, and non-violently claiming personal power.

Learning Activities

Locate and read the two articles above to see how nurses have used Rogers's work.

1. Answer the following questions about Rogers's theory:
   a. What aspects of humanity are explored in the theory?
   b. What are the central concepts that form the basis of the theory?
   c. Is there an overall theme that governs perceptions of the central concepts?
   d. How might the propositions expressed in this theory affect everyday nursing practice?
   e. Does the theory resonate with your own experience?
2. Perform an Internet search using the phrase *Hubble Space Telescope* to find stunning photographs of outer space taken from the Hubble Space Telescope. Print your favorite photo to represent Rogers's theory and share it with classmates.
3. Find websites or journal articles about Rogers's theory. Words to use when performing a search might include:
   - Martha Rogers
   - Unitary Human Beings
   - Rogerian

References

Biley, F. C. (2002). Nursing for the new millennium: Martha Rogers and the science of unitary human beings. *Theoria: Journal of Nursing Theory*, 9(3), 19–22.

Cowling, W. R. (1990). A template for nursing practice. In E. A. M. Barret (Ed.), *Visions of Rogers' science-based nursing* (pp. 45–65). New York, NY: National League for Nursing Press.

George, J. B. (2002). *Nursing theories: The base for professional nursing practice*. Upper Saddle River, NJ: Prentice Hall.

Rogers, M. E. (1966). Doctoral education in nursing. *Nursing Forum*, 5(2), 75–82.

Rogers, M. E. (1994). Educating the nurse for the future. In V. M. Malinski & E. A. M. Barrett (Eds.). *Martha Rogers: Her life and work* (pp. 61–68). Philadelphia, PA: F. A. Davis.

Tomey, A. M., & Alligood, M. R. (2002). *Nursing theorists and their work* (5th ed.). St. Louis, MO: Mosby.

Margaret Newman's Health as Expanding Consciousness

Margaret Newman was born in Memphis, Tennessee, in 1933. She earned a Behavioral Sciences and Health Education degree in home economics and English from Baylor University in Texas in 1954. After caring for her mother during a terminal illness, Newman decided to become a nurse. She earned a Bachelor of Science degree in nursing from the University of Memphis in 1962 and a Master of Science degree in nursing from the University of California in San Francisco in 1964. In 1971, she earned a doctorate in nursing science and rehabilitation from New York University. Newman taught at the University of Tennessee, New York University, and Pennsylvania State University. She retired from the University of Minnesota in 1996. She received many awards for nursing leadership and scholarship.

Newman's Health as Expanding Consciousness was influenced by Martha Rogers (Tomey & Alligood, 2002). Newman (2003) wrote:

The theory of health as expanding consciousness stems from Rogers' theory of Unitary Human Beings. Rogers' assumptions regarding patterning of persons in interaction with the environment are basic to the view that consciousness is a manifestation of an evolving pattern of person–environment interaction. . . . Consciousness includes not only the cognitive and affective awareness normally associated with consciousness, but also the interconnectedness of the entire living system, which includes physiochemical maintenance and growth processes as well as the immune system. This pattern of information, which is the consciousness of the system, is part of a larger, undivided pattern of an expanding universe.

Implicit in Newman's theory is the assumption that human beings have the following characteristics (George, 2002; Marchione, 1993):

- Are open energy systems
- Are in continual interconnectedness with a universe of open systems (environment)
- Are continuously active in evolving their own pattern of the whole (health)
- Are intuitive as well as affective cognitive beings
- Are capable of abstract thinking as well as sensation
- Are more than the sum of their parts

According to Newman (2003), when the concept of health is viewed as a wholistic pattern, illness is an expression emanating from the interaction between the client and the environment. When nurses view illness in this way, the usual focus on treatment of symptoms shifts to a focus on pattern recognition. Illness is viewed as part of the organizing process of expanding consciousness. One of the primary roles of the nurse becomes to help patients recognize and positively address their own patterns.

The focus of Newman's approach for nurses is to

- Attend to the "we" in a human-to-human exchange rather than viewing the other person as an object outside of ourselves
- Attend to the meaning of the whole rather than the "fixing" of a part or the sum of the parts
- Process the experience of interaction in partnership with the client
- Cultivate compassionate mutual consciousness rather than manipulation, or control, of another person's behavior
- Mindfully attend to the here and now (the moment) rather than try to identify past causes or possible future effects (George, 2002)

Newman skillfully weaves the elusive threads of this approach together with her words. About individuals, families, and communities, Newman (2000) says this:

> When we begin to think of ourselves as centers of consciousness (patterns of energy) within an overall pattern of expanding consciousness, we can begin to see what we sense of our lives is part of a much larger whole. First the pattern of consciousness that is the person; then broadening the focus, the pattern of consciousness that is the family and physical surroundings; then the pattern that is the community, the person's larger environmental affiliations, such as work or school; and ultimately the pattern of the world. (p. 24)

Health is a process of expanding consciousness. Humans are uniquely capable of gaining insight into their own patterns of life and health. All experiences related to health, illness, and death are part of the experience of progressing to a higher level of consciousness (Newman, 2000).

Nurses intervene and provide care by forming a partnership with the client. Partnerships include trust and immediacy and result in each participant reaching a higher level of consciousness (Newman, 2000).

Here is one way to visualize Newman's Health as Expanding Consciousness: envision a nurse and a client in a room standing a few feet away from one another. Each person is surrounded and permeated by light. Unique layers of different colored lights are moving around, within, and through each person. As the nurse and client shift toward and then away from one another in the course of an authentic caring exchange, the layers of color surrounding each person become mixed, creating new colors at every interchange. Ripples of soft light emanate from the doorway as people pass by or linger to convey greetings. The success of the exchange between nurse and client is apparent when the layers of light surrounding each gently expand outward to mingle yet further with each other and the surrounding light.

Theory in Action

Nursing theories are meant to stimulate and support knowledge development related to effectively exploring, predicting, describing, defining, and (sometimes) controlling nursing phenomena. Newman's work stresses wholism and nurse–patient collaboration. Nurses have the opportunity to empower patients by helping them gain insight into their own patterns of life and health. The two publications listed below, which are electronically accessible in the major databases, demonstrate Newman's theory in action:

MacNeil, J. M. (2012). The complexity of living with hepatitis C: A Newman perspective. *Nursing Science Quarterly*, 25, 261–266. doi:10.1177/0894318412447567

This article presents a qualitative study in which Newman's theory was utilized to explore patterns and meanings related to living with hepatitis C. Identified patterns included *struggling to overcome, transcending the illness,* and *wanting to give back.*

Awa, M., & Yamashita, M. (2008). Persons' experience of HIV/AIDS in Japan: Application of Margaret Newman's theory. *International Nursing Review*, 55(4), 454–461. doi: 10.1111/j.1466-7657.2008.00658.x

This article describes a qualitative study of the lived experience of five men living with HIV/AIDS in Japan. Identified evolving patterns included *self-conscious of own sexual orientation, chaos, stagnation, turning point,* and *regaining a new identity.*

Learning Activities

Locate and read the two articles listed above to see how nurses have used Newman's work.

1. Answer the following questions about Newman's theory:
   a. What aspects of humanity are explored in the theory?
   b. What are the central concepts that form the basis of the theory?
   c. Is there an overall theme that governs perceptions of the central concepts?
2. How might the propositions expressed in this theory affect everyday nursing practice?
3. Does the theory resonate with your own experience?
4. Perform an Internet search using the phrase *Hubble Space Telescope* to find stunning photographs of outer space taken from the Hubble Space Telescope. Print your favorite photo to represent Newman's theory and share it with classmates.

5. Find websites or journal articles about Newman's theory. Words to use when performing a search might include:
   - Margaret Newman
   - Health as Expanding Consciousness

References

George, J. B. (2002). *Nursing theories: The base for professional nursing practice.* Upper Saddle River, NJ: Prentice Hall.

Marchione, J. (1993). *Margaret Newman: Health as expanding consciousness.* Newbury Park, CA: Sage.

Newman, M. (2000). *Health as expanding consciousness* (2nd ed.). Sudbury, MA: Jones and Bartlett Publishing and National League for Nursing.

Newman, M. (2003). Overview. Health as Expanding Consciousness. Retrieved from http://healthasexpandingconsciousness.org/home/index.php?option=com_content&task=view&id=5&Itemid=6

Tomey, A. M., & Alligood, M. R. (2002). *Nursing theorists and their work* (5th ed.). St. Louis, MO: Mosby.

Rosemarie Rizzo Parse's Theory of Human Becoming

Rosemarie Rizzo Parse was born in on July 28, 1938, in Pittsburgh, Pennsylvania (Ancestry.com, 2015; Reed & Shearer, 2009). Parse grew up in Castle Shannon, Pennsylvania, in a warm and supportive family. Her father was the oldest of seven children and worked with his father as a lamplighter and later became a borough manager for Castle Shannon. Her mother was a homemaker and a very active member of the local Catholic church. Parse has two siblings, an older sister, Nancy, who is also a nurse, and a brother named Frank. Her family emphasized education and the arts, and Parse took piano and dancing lessons while growing up. Parse was raised a strict Catholic and describes her childhood as wonderful. Parse states that she enjoyed school and was a very good student.

After graduating from a Catholic high school, she attended Duquesne University in Pittsburgh, where she earned her bachelor's degree in nursing. Against the advice of the dean and faculty at Duquesne, she accepted a fellowship and immediately went on to work on her master's degree in nursing at the University of Pittsburgh. When she graduated in 2 years from Pitt, according to her husband, John Parse, she became the youngest person in the United States to hold a master's degree in nursing. She went on to earn a doctorate from the University of Pittsburgh while teaching at her alma mater,

Duquesne. At Duquesne, she became the first woman elected to chair the faculty senate and the first dean of nursing to hold a doctorate (Alligood, Krivicich, Kramer, Erickson, & Mishel, 2008).

Parse served as dean of nursing at Duquesne from 1983 to 1993 and professor and Niehoff chair at Loyola University from 1993 to 2006. Since 2007, she has served as a consultant and visiting scholar at New York University. Parse founded the Institute of Human Becoming and the journal *Nursing Science Quarterly*, and she still serves as the journal's editor. At the *Nursing Science Quarterly*, Parse oversees a very important venue for the discussion and debate of nursing research and theory. More information about Parse can be found at *the* International Consortium of Parse Scholars (http://www.humanbecoming.org) and Discovery International (http://www.discoveryinternationalonline.com).

The Theory of Human Becoming

Parse's theoretical development originated from the values her parents instilled in her in childhood. The theory grew over time. The dignity of every human being was very important to her, and she described the conflict she experienced when trying to understand and use the biophysical-medical model as a framework for practice. So, she began searching for a model that matched her specific worldview, which led to the creation of her own nursing theory.

Parse's Theory of Human Becoming was known as the man/living/health model when it was first published in 1981. In 1992, the theory's name was changed to Human Becoming to better reflect its focus on humankind without gender distinction. Parse's theory is similar to that of Martha Rogers's theory of Unitary Human Beings, and both are often referred to as simultaneity theories because they focus on a unitary human where the whole is different from the sum of its parts and cannot be understood by knowledge of the parts.

Parse read widely in the field of psychology and philosophy in addition to nursing and readily acknowledges the philosophical sources of her theory as being Martha Rogers's Science of Unitary Human Beings and the existential philosophers Søren Kierkegaard, Franz Kafka, Martin Heidegger, Jean-Paul Sartre, and Maurice Merleau-Ponty (Reed, Shearer, & Nicoll, 2004).

Also, during the 1960s and 1970s when Parse studied at Duquesne University, the university was regarded by some as the center of the existential-phenomenological movement, and Parse was heavily influenced by this school of thought while she studied there (Parse, 1981).

Basic Beliefs/Assumptions

Many of Parse's major assumptions come from Rogers's Science of Unitary Human Beings (1970, 1992) and the existential philosophers. Parse believes that human beings are intentional; they choose and assign meaning to events, and like Rogers, she believes that human beings cannot be reduced to component parts and be fully understood. Parse's main belief is that human beings coauthor their becoming along with the universe, cocreating distinct patterns. Parse also believes that human beings have free choice and cocreate health together with the universe. Therefore, the human must be viewed as an expert on his or her own health and lived experiences (Parse, 1995). Parse's use of "co" means together with and is used extensively in her work.

Parse's theory includes nine assumptions, which are as follows:

1. The human is coexisting while coconstituting rhythmic patterns in the universe.
2. The human is an open being, freely choosing meaning in situation, bearing responsibility for decisions.
3. The human is a living unity continuously coconstituting patterns of relating.
4. The human is transcending multidimensionally with the possibilities.
5. Becoming is an open process experienced by the human.
6. Becoming is a rhythmically coconstituting human–universe process.
7. Becoming is the human's pattern of relating value priorities.
8. Becoming is an intersubjective process of transcending with the possibilities.
9. Becoming is human evolving. (Parse, 1998, pp. 5–6)

Parse's theory includes three assumptions about human becoming:

1. Human becoming is freely choosing personal meaning in a situation in the intersubjective process of relating value priorities.

2. Human becoming is cocreating rhythmic patterns of relating in open process with the universe.
3. Human becoming is cotranscending multidimensionally with the emerging possible. (Parse, 1992, p. 38)

The four main components of Parse's theory are the mutual process of the human universe, the coconstitution of health, the multidimensional meanings the indivisible human gives to being and becoming, and the human's freedom in situations to choose alternative paths of becoming.

Parse asserts that the human is coexisting while coconstituting rhythmic patterns with the environment. Coexistence means that humans are not alone in any "dimension of becoming" (Parse, 1998, p. 17). To create her nine assumptions, Parse pulled from Rogers's principles of helicy, integrality, and resonancy; her concepts of energy field, openness, pattern, and four dimensionality; as well as major constructs found in existential philosophy (Reed et al., 2004). The Theory of Human Becoming is the only nursing theory that regards paradoxes as an integral part of the human experience. Paradoxes are normal in life and, according to Parse, should not be viewed as a problem to be solved.

Parse's theory is based on three main themes or concepts entitled meaning, rhythmicity, and transcendence. Each of these themes gives rise to additional concepts where structuring meaning relates to the concepts of imagining, valuing, and languaging; the concept of rhythmicity relates to revealing–concealing, enabling–limiting, and connecting–separating; and the concept of transcendence relates to powering, originating, and transforming.

Principles

Parse outlines three principles in her theory that she indicates flow from her theoretical assumptions. Each of the three principles has three component concepts. The three principles are as follows:

Principle 1: Structuring meaning multidimensionally is cocreating reality through the languaging of valuing and imaging (Parse, 1998, p. 35). Component concepts are imaging, valuing, and languaging.

Principle 2: Cocreating rhythmic patterns of relating is living the paradoxic unity of revealing–concealing and enabling–limiting while connecting–separating (Parse, 1998, p. 42). Component concepts are revealing–concealing, enabling–limiting, and connecting–separating.

Principle 3: Cotranscending with the possible is powering unique ways of originating in the process of transforming (Parse, 1998, p. 46). Component concepts are powering, originating, and transforming.

Structuring meaning explains that humans choose the meaning of their own realities, and the choosing that occurs is not always a conscious undertaking. This explains why people often lack insight into their behavior. Imaging, valuing, and languaging are component concepts within the principle of structuring. Imaging is how a person sees his or her own reality, valuing is the process by which a person confirms his or her beliefs, and languaging is the process by which humans express their reality. Languaging can occur with words or symbols or by using nonverbal signals, movement, and so forth (Parse, 1981, 1998).

Cocreating is the second principle and involves the process that humans use to express their personal values and meanings through the creation of patterns. Cocreation means that people live in rhythm with the universe. It is about choices, connections, and letting go. The concepts embedded in cocreating are revealing–concealing, enabling–limiting, and connecting–separating. Revealing–concealing is the process humans use to show or hide their personal evolution or becoming. It involves how much we want to share about ourselves with others. Enabling–limiting refers to the opportunities or restrictions that occur daily. Humans are confronted with opportunities every moment, and choices are made whether to act upon the chance or not. Enabling–limiting is about making choices and living with the consequences of actions. Connecting–separating is a description of the creation of patterns through the processes of connecting and separating with people, things, and places. Connecting and separating is about joining with and separating from something (Parse, 1981, 1998).

Cotranscending is about humans engaging with and choosing how to be and the attitudes and approaches they select. Powering, originating, and transforming are the concepts that make up the principle of cotranscending. Powering is the concept that relates the struggle humans display when confronted with hardships and threats. Powering is a push–pull process that is always occurring. Originating is about the uniqueness of humans. Humans seek to be original and stand apart from others and yet at the same time feel the need to blend in. This sense of being unique and needing to be like others causes certainty and uncertainty. Transforming is the third concept in cotranscending and is about creating deliberate change and the way humans view themselves. Transforming is a continuous process of evolution as humans seek to understand the changes occurring (Parse, 1981, 1998).

Nursing

Parse does not write about nursing as a concept in her theory; however, she refers to the core of nursing science and nursing's focus of concern as the human–universe–health process, which, according to Parse, is the basic interrelationship of the human, the universe, and health (Parse, 1992). Parse believes that quality of life is the goal of nursing. The belief that human beings are free to choose is fundamental to the practice of nursing with all actions focused on guiding humans toward ways of being, finding meaning, and choosing ways of cocreating their own health (Parse, 1995, 1998). Parse also writes about requirements that she believes are essential for nursing practice, which are the following:

- Possessing the knowledge and use of nursing frameworks and theories
- Offering of self
- Valuing others
- Respecting differences
- Taking accountability for one's actions
- Desiring to experience and test that which is new and unknown
- Connecting with others
- Being proud of oneself
- Liking what one does
- Recognizing the joy and struggles in living
- Appreciating mystery and newness
- Being competent
- Having a willingness to rest and begin again (Parse, 1989)

Human–Universe–Health Process

According to Parse, human, universe, and health are concepts that cannot be viewed separately, and although they can be described individually, they are always linked together (Parse, 1990, 1996, 1998). Parse (1989) refers to health as a "cocreated process of becoming as experienced and described by the person, family and community" (p. 11). Health is a way of being in the world—not a continuum with health and illness at opposite ends but rather a day-to-day way of being. Health is a personal commitment with ebbs and flows.

Human beings can be described as intentional, knowing beings who are involved with their world, open to their world and cocreating meaning in multidimensional mutual process with the universe. This mutual process with the universe can be recognized by patterns of relating and the ability to freely choose. Parse believes that human beings have responsibility for their health. Parse views the universe as the world and those who occupy spaces along with others who freely choose to be in the situation (Parse, 1998). Like Rogers, Parse sees the human and the environment or universe as mutually and simultaneously interrelated and believes that the human–universe–health process is more than the sum of its parts and health is ever changing (Parse, 1987).

Summary

Parse's theory of human becoming is considered a grand theory that focuses on the irreducibility of human beings and the interrelationship between human beings and the universe. Although complex and somewhat difficult to understand because of the terminology and the abstractness of her concepts, Parse's writing offers a framework with which to view the patterns of human lived experiences. The perspective brought to nursing by the Human Becoming Theory is a very important one with human beings viewed as intentional, with the right to freely choose and more than the sum of the component parts. No doubt as more and more nurses use the theory in practice and in research, the Theory of Human Becoming will continue to offer a perspective of possibilities.

Theory in Action

Nursing theories are meant to stimulate and support knowledge development related to effectively exploring, predicting, describing, defining, and (sometimes) controlling nursing phenomena. Parse's work reflects interconnectivity, wholism, and human autonomy. The two historic publications listed below, which are electronically accessible in the major databases, demonstrate Parse's theory in action:

Relf, M. V. (1997). Illuminating meaning and transforming issues of spirituality in HIV and AIDS: An application of Parse's Theory of Human Becoming. *Holistic Nursing Practice*, 12(1), 1–8. doi:10.1097/00004650-199710000-00003

In this article, the author explores the concept of spirituality in nursing care with a focus on patients with HIV disease. Nursing strategies to support patient spirituality are proposed within the framework of Parse's Theory of Human Becoming.

Janes, N. M., & Wells, D. L. (1997). Elderly patients' experiences with nurses guided by Parse's Theory of Human Becoming. *Clinical Nursing Research*, 6, 205–222. doi:10.1177/105477389700600302

This article presented a study in which elderly patients described their experiences of being cared for by nurses who based their practices on Parse's Theory of Human Becoming. Three themes emerged: *coming together for instrumental tasks, nurses being there for patients,* and *nurses' pleasing way.* The authors concluded that results signified patients felt cared for and looked after.

Learning Activities

Locate and read the two articles listed above to see how nurses have used Parse's work.

1. Choose one of Parse's concepts, such as meaning, valuing, languaging, or revealing–concealing, and explain how it might be used to interpret a client's behavior.
2. Explain how denial often seen in clients with alcoholism might be interpreted using Parse's concepts.

3. Suggest some nursing interventions that would be consistent with Parse's theory and in what type of care scenario they might be used.

4. Discuss one idea or concept expressed by Parse that caused you to think more deeply about a client situation you might have encountered. How would your approach to your client have been different if viewed through Parse's Theory of Human Becoming?

References

Alligood, M. R., Krivicich, D., Kramer, A. S., Erickson, H. C., & Mishel, M. H. (2008). *The nurse theorists: Portraits of excellence* (Vol. 2). [Video recording]. Athens, OH: FITNE.

Ancestry.com. (2015). U.S. Public Record Index, Vol. 2. [database online]. Provo, UT: USA Ancestry.com Operations, Inc.

Parse, R. R. (1981). *Man-living-health: A theory of nursing*. New York, NY: John Wiley and Sons.

Parse, R. R. (1987). *Nursing science: Major paradigms, theories, and critiques*. Philadelphia, PA: W. B. Saunders.

Parse, R. R. (1989). Essentials for practicing the art of nursing. *Nursing Science Quarterly*, 2, 111.

Parse, R. R. (1990). Health: A personal commitment. *Nursing Science Quarterly*, 3, 136–140.

Parse, R. R. (1992). Human becoming: Parse's theory of nursing. *Nursing Science Quarterly*, 5, 35–42.

Parse, R. R. (1995). *Illuminations: The human becoming theory in practice and research*. New York, NY: National League for Nursing.

Parse, R. R. (1996). The human becoming: Challenges in practice and research. *Nursing Science Quarterly*, 9, 55–60.

Parse, R. R. (1998). *The human becoming school of thought: A perspective for nurses and other health professionals*. Thousand Oaks, CA: Sage.

Reed, P. G., & Shearer, N. B. C. (2009). *Perspectives on nursing theory* (5th ed.). Phildelphia, PA: Lippincott Williams & Wilkins.

Reed, P. G., Shearer, N. B. C., & Nicoll, L. H. (2004). *Perspectives on nursing theory* (4th ed.). Philadelphia, PA: Lippincott Williams & Wilkins.

Rogers, M. E. (1970). *An introduction to the theoretical basis of nursing*. Philadelphia: Davis.

Rogers, M. E. (1992). Nursing science and the space age. *Nursing Science Quarterly*, 5, 27–34.

Resources

Discovery International: http://www.discoveryinternationalonline.com

International Consortium of Parse Scholars: http://www.humanbecoming.org

Loyola University Monroe Library: Dawtrey, Adam. (2012). Pros parse past year's pedigree. *Daily Variety*, 315(4), 26.

Interview with Dr. Parse

Nursing Science Quarterly: http://nsq.sagepub.com/

Conclusion

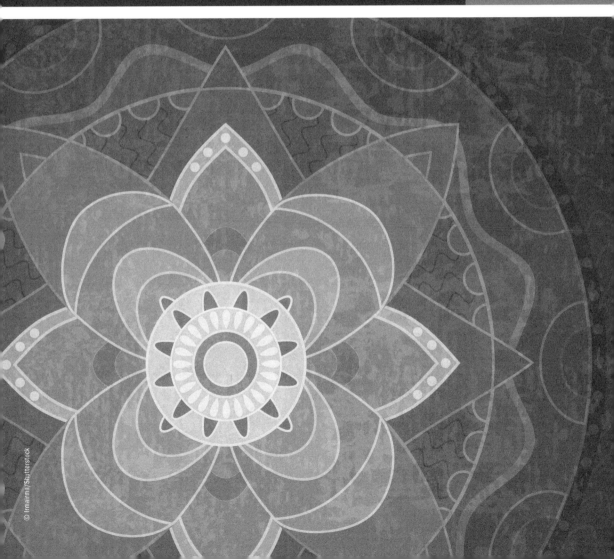

Further Development of Nursing Theory

Theories about nursing are as varied as nurses themselves. Some nurse leaders believe that development of theory supporting evidence-based practice is where future focus should be (Evers, 2001). Many questions remain that must be formally explored and answered regarding effective nursing practice (Evers, 2001). Other nurses believe that "nursing theories are needed that have social justice as their goal" (Drevdahl, 1999, p. 1). These nurses believe that, in the future, broad social issues will supersede other nursing concerns and create the need for theories that address environmental problems, global poverty, diminishing health status, and ethnic and religious conflicts (Drevdahl, 1999). Still others value the development of theories that explore what it means to inhabit a human body and experience issues associated with health and wellness (sentience) (Wilde, 1999). Theories are also being developed that are based on the notion that *caring* is the central concept that makes nursing a unique profession (Watson, 2003). Probably the roots of theory development in nursing began with Florence Nightingale during the Crimean War in Turkey when she hypothesized about the connection between hygiene and health and began to systematically record her observations to test these associations (Nightingale, 1992).

There are many different kinds of theories because nurses provide care to human beings and human beings are multifaceted, having physical, mental, spiritual, psychological, social, and existential elements. One theory, or one type of theory, could not begin to fully describe all that is nursing. Also, every nurse that seeks to describe nursing practice through the creation of a theory has a slightly different vantage point from any other nurse. There will always be a wide array of theories that describe the practice of nursing.

Unfortunately, there is a general sense that, within the nursing ranks, two distinct theoretical camps exist. One camp values scientific, structured inquiry over all other methods of exploring and clarifying what nursing *is* and what nurses *do*. The other camp values narrative, personalized inquiry (Glazer, 2000). This division is not necessary because both kinds of theory arise from different aspects of nursing practice, and both aspects are needed in nursing.

Effective nursing practice requires highly structured technical knowledge and action based on scientific inquiry and theory generation. Effective nursing practice *also* requires less structured, but equally valid, knowledge and action regarding mental, spiritual, psychological, social, and existential human experience based on narrative, personalized inquiry, and theory building. The combination of both kinds of theory forms a complete picture of the profession, and neither approach could begin to fully express all that nursing *is*.

Nursing actions are practical in nature; thus, theory should guide and clarify actual practice. This creates a need for scholarly theory that has the potential to improve practice. As Cash (2001) states, "Because nursing is a practical activity, theory has to be a guide to practice, not an end in itself. In other words, the concepts to be clarified have to be relevant to clinical practice in some way and conclusions reached lead to some new or changed action" (p. 2). All of the theories explored in this text have the power to change nursing practice on some level, depending on how and in what situation the theory is used.

Many nursing theories have their roots in theories and models originating in the sociological, behavioral, and biological sciences. Before nursing theories were created or in wide use, nurse researchers based their work on nonnursing models and frameworks. Contemporary nurses may still find conceptual models and frameworks, such as social exchange theory and others, appropriate for the foundation of their practice or research (Lee, Hann, Yang, & Fawcett, 2011; Shieh, Tung, & Liang, 2012).

In clarifying the need for a variety of nursing theories, a common childhood story comes to mind: one day, the king of a small kingdom went hunting with the fire chief. While they were gone, the king's palace caught fire due to an unfortunate kitchen mishap. Because the fire chief was out hunting with the king, the volunteer fire department did not mobilize to put the fire out, and the whole palace burned to the ground. Upon the king's return, it was mandated that every adult in the kingdom should abandon their chosen profession and become a firefighter so that the palace would never burn down again. After a week of no bakery goods, no fresh produce, no clean laundry or dishes, no babysitters, no school teachers, no construction workers, and no police, the king realized that it takes more than firefighters to effectively run a kingdom. He mandated that everyone return to their old jobs. The moral of the story: it takes all kinds to effectively run a kingdom (or, in this case, the nursing profession).

The key to progress with respect to theory generation lies in the ability of nurses and nursing leaders to appreciate the unique value in a variety of approaches, even when some approaches do not resonate with every nurse. In this way, the knowledge base in the profession will continue to grow, reflecting the richness and diversity found in the nursing ranks and nursing practice.

As the profession of nursing continues to evolve, nursing theories will also evolve. More middle-range theories will be created to clarify effective nursing approaches in specific clinical areas, and there will be further clarification of how to apply nursing grand theories and philosophies. Older theories will be expanded, revisited, and explored for relevancy to today's nursing practice, and new theories will be created. Newer theories will evolve based on current practice concerns and questions that are influenced by the current healthcare and general social climate. One of the most valuable aspects of theory development in nursing is the ongoing thought, dialogue, and variety precipitated by the process. Another valuable aspect is that the continued development of theory will lead to better-informed practice for all nurses.

Learning Activities

1. Recall the background information you have read about each one of the nurse theorists. Which theorists do you think had the most interesting reason for developing her nursing theory? Be prepared to share and defend your answer and rationale.

2. We have finished reviewing all the nursing theories now. Which one "speaks" to you and why? If none of them do, why not? What is missing? What would it take for one to make sense to you?

3. Nurses are free to choose a nursing theory or nonnursing theorist as the basis for their practice or research. As a general rule, do you think one is better for the profession? If so, which one and why? If not, why not?

References

Cash, K. (2001). Theory as resistance. *Nursing Philosophy*, 2, 1–3.

Drevdahl, D. (1999). Sailing beyond: Nursing theory and the person. *Advances in Nursing Science*, 21(4), 1–13.

Evers, G. C. M. (2001). Naming nursing: Evidence-based nursing. *Nursing Diagnosis*, 12(4), 137–141.

Glazer, S. (2000). Postmodern nursing. *Public Interest*, 140, 3–16.

Lee, H., Hann, H. W., Yang, J., & Fawcett, J. (2011). Recognition and management of HIV infection in a social context. *Journal of Cancer Education*, 26, 516–521.

Nightingale, F. (1992). *Notes on nursing: What it is and what it is not*. Philadelphia, PA: Lippincott Williams, & Wilkins.

Shieh, S. C., Tung, H. S., & Liang, S. Y. (2012). Social support as influencing primary family caregiver burden in Taiwanese patients with colorectal cancer. *Journal of Nursing Scholarship*, 44(30), 223–231.

Watson, J. (2003). Dr. Jean Watson biography. Retrieved from http://www.ucdenver.edu/academics/colleges/nursing/programs-admissions/doctoral-programs/doctor-philosophy/caringscience/Pages/Jean-Watson-Biography.aspx

Wilde, M. H. (1999). Why embodiment now? *Advances in Nursing Science*, 22(2), 25–38.

Use of Information Technology by Nurse Theorists

More than 150 years ago, Nightingale wrote her thoughts with pen and ink by candlelight. Her thoughts were compiled into a small book called *Notes on Nursing*, and she began the profession of nursing (Nightingale, 1859). Nightingale's *Notes on Nursing* was reprinted in 1992 and has been widely disseminated. She was the earliest nurse theorist leaving instructions for gathering nursing knowledge and evidence and establishing linkages for improving patient care (Nightingale, 1992). It took almost 100 years for nursing to embrace the need for nursing theory and to begin again.

In 1900, the *American Journal of Nursing* was the first formal method of communicating nursing knowledge to nurses who were lucky enough to have access to it (Kalisch & Kalisch, 1995). Full-text journal articles are now available online any time on virtually any computer, as needed. Today, the creation, development, refinement, and dissemination of knowledge are radically different from just 20 years ago, and certainly different from 125 years ago. This radical change has occurred in large part because of computer and Internet technology.

With global travel, telecommunications, information technology, auto-translate, and the Internet, the boundaries of space, time, geography, and language have greatly diminished the barriers that nurse theorists faced in the twentieth century. Today, because of current technology, it is possible for almost any student to ask a major, living theorist, or an expert on a theorist, a question about a theory and receive an answer without ever leaving his or her living room. Nurses with similar interests in a theory now have the opportunity to connect with colleagues around the world who are interested in the same theorist. The Internet gives nurses opportunities that they would otherwise never have. Meeting and learning from participation in online communities and discussions further the understanding of nursing theory and application and utilization by nurses in practice.

Current Uses of Technology

Nursing theory entered cyberspace in the mid- to late 1980s and early to mid-1990s when nurses began using email and listservs, or "cyber circles," and websites to communicate. The use of information technology resulted in a paradigm shift in the dissemination of information and in relationships among theorists.

One of the unique characteristics of the Internet is its ability to connect millions of people instantaneously at any time. Certainly, books, journals, and some audiovisual media have the ability to transmit knowledge, but they do not have the ability to facilitate "community" like the Internet and media that use the Internet do. This "connectedness" has the potential to create a community that is not limited by space, time, geography, or sociopolitical issues. Connectedness is limited only by one's ability to access the Internet. The ability to connect has allowed nurses to find others with whom they share common theory and research interests. Through online discussions, chats, blogs, and listservs, nurses who have ideas and questions about theories have the opportunity to seek feedback, support, and funding ideas. Not only do online discussions provide access to new colleagues but also computer-mediated chats allow individuals who are timid and hesitant to speak up in groups to ask questions they would never speak in public (Deering & Eichelberger, 2002).

Listservs were one of the original communication tools used by groups of nurse theorists. One of the oldest listservs is Parse-L, which was created on February 4, 1993, by Pat Lyon. It is an international discussion forum and information exchange network for Parse's Theory of Human Becoming. Dr. Parse monitors the list and occasionally responds to questions. Students often sign on to ask questions for theory assignments. In general, theory listservs are quite manageable and do not have as much traffic as other nursing listservs. Dr. Imogene King has a blog where devotees or students with questions can post on the blog and have a King expert respond.

Nursing Theory Websites

The most common type of online communication used by nurse theorists remains their websites. In some cases, nurse theorists host their own websites; in most cases, organizations formed by nurses who study or conduct research using a particular theory host the theory's website.

There are two types of theory websites: compilation sites and content sites. Compilation sites are composite sites of links where visitors can go to find connections to pages on various nursing theories. In addition, these sites may offer various other theory-related links, such as those for theory conferences, textbooks, email addresses of theorists, and other theory-related sites.

In contrast, content sites are devoted to an individual theorist or theory. Most theorists have a website devoted to their theory; however, some do not have any information on the Web. If you have an interest in developing Web material for a theorist who does not have a website, please contact Dr. Lisa Wright Eichelberger at lisaeichelberger@clayton.edu.

Compilation Sites

The Nursing Theory Page (http://www.sandiego.edu/nursing/research/nursing-theory-research.php/) is the original nursing theory compilation site on the Internet. It is a collaborative effort of an international group of dedicated individuals committed to sharing nursing theory within the profession. The group seeks to develop a complete collection of resources about nursing theories used throughout the world. The project began on May 21, 1996, and has played a very important part in the advancement of nursing theory. Dr. Judy Norris of the University of Alberta was the founding webmaster and served in that capacity until May 2003, when she retired. At that time, the webmaster duties were transferred to the Hahn School of Nursing and Health Sciences at the University of San Diego.

The Eichelberger Nursing Theory website (http://www.clayton.edu/nursing/Nursing-Theory) began November 1, 1996, as a part of a class assignment in Dr. Lisa Wright Eichelberger's Nursing Theory class at Clayton State University (CSU), Atlanta, Georgia, when students Tommy Thomas and Carolyn Stewart were dismayed at the lack of information available about nursing theorists on the World Wide Web. Since 1997, Dr. Eichelberger has been the webmaster for this compilation site and often responds to emails from students from all over the world who ask for information about different theorists. Unfortunately, there are still theorists for whom no information exists on the Web. (See the CSU site for a list of theorists without a website.) The Eichelberger Nursing Theory site has received more than 1.5 million hits since its inception, indicating the level of interest in information about nursing theory on the Internet.

Content Sites

Most nurse theorists have some sort of Web presence, whether it be a professionally developed website or a link to a simple biography or obituary. As with all content on websites, addresses change and links break, so it is important to notify a webmaster of inactive links. A few theorists have email addresses and can be reached with a simple email. Even if the theorist is deceased, individuals who are experts or historians with expert knowledge of the nurse theorist often are available and willing to assist others in learning about a particular nurse theorist.

Florence Nightingale, for example, has one of the most extensive Web presences of any theorist and a bulletin board devoted to her. Nightingale has quite a fan in "Country Joe" McDonald, who sponsored and served as webmaster for one of Nightingale's most interesting websites since November 1996. McDonald, a Vietnam veteran and musician who performed at the famous 1969 Woodstock Festival, has also recorded songs about Nightingale. McDonald's songs about Nightingale can be heard on the Nightingale site as well (http://scienceofcaring.ucsf.edu/profiles-nursing/without-nurses-i-don%E2%80%99t-know-where-f-we-would-be) retrieved from the web April 10th, 2015.

In 2003, McDonald reported receiving approximately 300 hits per day during the school year, many from school-age children (J. McDonald, personal communication, June 8, 2003). According to Tom Weller, analytics manager for the

"Country Joe" McDonald Nightingale website, from March 2014 to March 2015, there was an average of 1,483 visits per month, or approximately 50 hits per day to the /nightingale/ folder entry page; this number does not include visits originating from an internal page such as nightingale/pledge.htm, which is a very popular page (personal communication, April 9, 2015).

One of the most exciting opportunities that the Internet provides is communication directly with a particular theorist. Some theory sites have blogs or bulletin boards where anyone can post a question and the nurse theorist or expert will answer it. Having the opportunity to ask the theorist or expert a question and receive a response is very exciting and helpful, particularly to students learning about theories.

Dissemination of Information

Nurses who are developing a new theory can use the Internet and the World Wide Web to introduce their theory to the nursing community at large and to connect with others who might wish to test the new theories. For a variety of reasons, it is sometimes very difficult to publish a book or have a manuscript published in a peer-reviewed journal, and the time lag between the conception of an idea and its publication can be quite lengthy. However, it is relatively simple and quick to publish an article on a website. This is both good and bad. It is good for the novice theorist who wishes to have a forum in which to present his or her work, but it is bad in the sense that the work may not be credible, clear, concise, valid, usable, generalizable, or reviewed by others. Just as with anything that is published on the Web, readers must evaluate the credibility of any new theory published online. When reviewing theory on the Web, remember to evaluate the source carefully. On the Web, at least 15 people will think that what you have said is fabulous (Weinberger, 2002).

When a theorist publishes a theory on the Web, many people read the theory and offer feedback. This feedback enables the theorist to revise to improve the theory. This exposure also creates opportunities for the theorist to locate others who share similar thoughts and interests. Through this exposure, collaborative situations often emerge. Kolcaba, who was developing her Theory of Comfort during 1988 to 1994, just as the Web was taking hold, used the Internet to communicate with Eichelberger about her theory as a way to disseminate information about the new theory.

Another example occurred with Dr. Sharon L. Van Sell of Texas Women's University, Houston, Texas, and Ioannis A. Kalofissudis of Greece and their Complexity Nursing Theory. In 2000, Van Sell found Kalofissudis's Holistic Conceptual Development Model of Nursing Science on the Web. Van Sell was very interested in Kalofissudis's theory because conceptually it was very similar to her theory of Nursing Knowledge and Practice. Van Sell traveled to Greece to discuss how they could expand their ideas and make them international in scope. They collaborated and "gave birth" to a new theory called the Complexity Nursing Theory. Without the Web, this new theory would most likely have never been developed. (I. Kalofissudis, personal communication, June 8, 2003). Since the creation of Van Sell and Kalofissudis's theory in 2000 and the publication of their eBook, approximately 50 peer-reviewed articles have been published using Complexity Theory as the conceptual basis (Sharon Van Sell, personal communication, April 10, 2015). Links to the Complexity Integration Theory eBook can be found at the Texas Women's University library. The Internet also led to contact being established among Kalofissudis, Van Sell, and Eichelberger, which in turn led to the sharing of information about the Complexity Integration Theory on Eichelberger's Theory Compilation website and an invitation to publish a chapter on Complexity Integration Theory in the third edition of this textbook.

Additionally, the coauthors of this textbook, Sitzman and Eichelberger, first connected online when Sitzman and her theory students, who were located in Utah, used Eichelberger's nursing theory website as a resource for Sitzman's nursing theory class. Sitzman contacted Eichelberger in Atlanta, Georgia, to discuss their mutual love of nursing theory. A collaboration was formed, and the decision to write a theory textbook was made in 2003.

Information technology and the Internet have dramatically changed the way nursing theorists organize, consult, and share information about theory, practice, research, and virtually every aspect of the domain of nursing. The use of information technology and the Internet by the nursing profession will continue to evolve. Online technology holds great potential for nurse theorists to assist in the generation, testing, and application of knowledge faster and more globally than ever before. It is, however, important to remember that technology is just a tool and the online community is what we make it. It is truly an exciting time to be a nurse theorist.

Theory in Action

The true test of theory comes from its use in practice. When a theory or framework is applied in the clinical setting, that is when it becomes evident whether the constructs and premises hold true and fit together. Below are two examples of clinical situations where researchers are testing the use of Van Sell and Kalofissudis's Complexity Integration Theory in practice.

Binner, M., Ross, D., & Browner, I. (2011). Chemotherapy-induced peripheral neuropathy: Assessment of oncology nurses' knowledge and practice. *Oncology Nursing Forum*, 38(4), 448–454.

This is a cross-sectional, exploratory study of 39 oncology nurses' practice behaviors regarding chemotherapy-induced peripheral neuropathy. Van Sell and Kalofissudis's Complexity Integration Theory is used as the theoretical framework to explain the level of knowledge and clinical practice behaviors.

Jeffery, F. D., Mutsch, K. S., & Knapp, L. (2014). Recognition of SIRS and sepsis among pediatric nurses. *Pediatric Nursing*, 40(6), 271–278.

The study was designed as a cross-sectional, quantitative, descriptive research study. Two hundred forty-two critical care nurses' knowledge level about pediatric patients' systematic inflammatory response syndrome (SIRS) was assessed and compared to corresponding treatment plans for patients with sepsis. Discrepancies were found between nurses' perceived level of knowledge and actual knowledge level.

Learning Activities

1. Imagine how nursing might have been different if Nightingale had had access to the Internet.
2. If Nightingale could have chosen to live in the 1800s or today, which do you think she would choose and why?
3. Discuss the types of listservs/discussion groups/blogs currently available on the Web for nurses interested in nursing theorists.
4. Formulate one question and post it on a nurse theorist's bulletin board or listserv. Share the responses that you receive with your classmates.

5. Discuss the possible reasons some nurse theorists do not have a presence on the Web. Why do you think some theorist have much more of an Internet presence than others? What does it take to create and maintain a site for a theorist?

References

Deering, C. G., & Eichelberger, L. W. (2002). Mirror mirror on the wall: Using online discussion groups to improve interpersonal skills. CIN: *Computer, Informatics, Nursing, 20*, 150–156.

Kalisch, P. A., & Kalisch, B. J. (1995). *The advance of American nursing* (3rd ed.). Philadelphia, PA: Lippincott Williams & Wilkins.

Nightingale, F. (1859). *Notes on nursing: What it is, and what it is not*. Philadelphia, PA: Edward Stern and Company.

Nightingale, F. (1992). *Notes on nursing: What it is and what it is not*. Philadelphia, PA: Lippincott Williams & Wilkins.

Weinberger, D. (2002). *Small pieces loosely joined: A unified theory of the Web*. Cambridge, MA: Perseus Publishing.

Twentieth Anniversary of Nursing Theory on the World Wide Web

Lisa Wright Eichelberger

Thinking of oneself as a pioneer is somewhat daunting and oftentimes associated with reaching a certain advanced age. The advanced age part was not something I particularly enjoyed considering. When I was approached about writing a chapter on pioneering nursing theory on the World Wide Web (WWW), I was somewhat hesitant, not quite seeing the value of such a chapter at first glance. However, after reflection, I agreed. And now, with the 20th anniversary of my website fast approaching, I have come to begin to understand the revolution that was and is the knowledge explosion of the Internet. The Internet has assisted the advancement of nursing theory and the creation of a worldwide community of nursing scholars like nothing else we have experienced.

Having a front-row seat to the comings and goings-on of nursing theory on the Internet has taught me a couple of things. The first lesson learned is that few inventions have caused a greater shift in our worldview than the Internet has, and, second, the lack of permanency of recorded information on the Web can be a major threat to our knowledge base. We have all experienced the Web phenomenon of "here today, gone tomorrow." So it is for those reasons that I have attempted to record a history of nursing theory on the Web and share with you some of my experiences as the webmaster of one of the first nursing theory websites. I feel very fortunate to have played a small part in facilitating access to nursing theory knowledge on the Web for those seeking to understand how nursing theory advances the profession of nursing.

The Beginning

I almost left nursing during the 1980s. I was a young nurse, armed with a master's degree, about to embark on doctoral study when I became very disillusioned with what I saw happening in nursing at the national level. You will recall from your study of nursing history that the late 1970s and early 1980s were a rather tumultuous time for the profession primarily because of the American Nurses Association's 1985 proposal looming on the horizon. The 1985 proposal referred to, of course, requiring a baccalaureate degree in nursing for entry into professional practice. Although this requirement has yet to become a reality, the proposal caused considerable turmoil and division within the profession for quite some time.

As a nurse educator in my 20s, I served as an associate director of a school of nursing, an opportunity and privilege few have today at such a young age. That leadership position afforded me the opportunity to foray into the national arena, where I quickly became disillusioned and discouraged with the nursing profession. I witnessed grown women yelling and screaming at one another during national educational meetings and using irrational and illogical arguments while debating entry into practice. This type of defeatist behavior and lack of vision on the part of nursing made me seriously consider leaving the profession. I was not sure that I wanted to continue to be a part of a profession that was so divided and whose leaders demonstrated such unreasonable and unprofessional behavior.

But during that time, I also had the good fortune to discover something else about nursing—the beauty and wisdom of nursing theory. I can honestly say that if it had not been for the study of nursing theory, I might not have remained in nursing. The disillusionment and discouragement that I was feeling in my professional life were overcome by the excitement and pure joy I found in studying the work of nurse theorists. I remained in nursing because of the intellectual challenge I encountered when analyzing nursing theory.

During my doctoral study at the University of Alabama at Birmingham, I discovered a completely new and different way of thinking when studying the work of nursing theorists. Martha Rogers's work was particularly intriguing and thought provoking for me. I remember thinking after reading Rogers's (1970) *Little Purple Book* and the *Tao of Physics* (Capra, 1975) how much nursing had to offer that was intellectually stimulating and thought provoking. And although a certain amount of craziness was demonstrated almost daily around me, I found a place where I could focus my thoughts and hopes.

My worldview changed after reading about Rogers's *Science of Unitary Man* (Rogers, 1970) as it was referred to at the time. Rogers later changed the name of her theory to the Science of Unitary Human Being. Rogers's theory, in particular, made me question everything about the way I viewed nursing and the world. It helped me to understand the complexities of the science that is nursing, and I rediscovered what I had originally loved about nursing. Rogers's *Science of Unitary Human Man* did that for me. While studying for my PhD at the University of Alabama at Birmingham, I was afforded the opportunity to personally meet and study with many of the early nurse theorists, and I was so inspired by them and their true pioneering thinking; it made me proud to be a nurse. In 1991, when I was a very young nurse, I was also privileged to have a private, one-on-one dinner with Virginia Henderson when she was 93 years old. For nearly 2 hours, she let me ask her anything and everything about her life and theory. I was in heaven.

So, I became a lover of theory, embracing it, using it, and relying on it to frame my approach to patient care. I turned inward, if you will, and switched my focus from the disorganization and confusion occurring at the national level of nursing to a focus on my views of nursing and how nursing theory could change one's entire approach to nursing practice and research. Nursing theory saved nursing for me, and I think it is for that reason that I have devoted so much of my personal time to advancing nursing theory on the Web.

The Web

Those of us who became nurses in the 1970s have experienced two revolutionary events in our careers—the development of AIDS and the development of the Internet. We can all remember starting IVs and attending deliveries without wearing gloves and spending hours in the basements of libraries gathering information and learning without the help of the Internet. I think most would agree that both occurrences have radically changed nursing.

Humans have always had the need to communicate with others, and so it is not hard to understand the success of the Web. The Internet is a worldwide system of interconnected networks and computers that allows us to communicate with one another in a very fast and immediate way that is not limited by proximity. But I think few in 1970 could have imagined our dependence on it today.

Although the exact timing, purpose, and development of what are known as the Web and the Internet can be debated, I think most would agree that the desire for resource sharing that occurred in the early 1970s was at the heart of this development. Not until the mid-1980s did the Web and email begin to be used for daily communications across communities.

Nursing Theory on the Web

If you study the evolution of the World Wide Web, it is easy to see the parallels with nursing theory evolution. The development of the Web mirrors the development of nursing theory as a whole, with the foundations of both laid in the 1800s and early 1900s, much work accomplished in the 1960s and 1970s, and huge advances made in the 1980s and 1990s.

The existence of nursing theory on the Internet began in the 1990s, but it is unclear which nurse theorist website was actually the first to be activated. Unfortunately, most of those who created nursing theory websites did not record when the site was first published. Unlike books with publication dates, many, if not most, of the theory websites have no traceable histories.

Even today, some nurse theorists currently have no Web presence. Twenty years ago, in 1996, when I first started working with nursing theory on the Web, I created a list of major nursing theorists who had no website and extended a standing offer to work with anyone who had the desire to create websites for these theorists. Unfortunately, the list of nursing theorists without websites has changed very little since 1996.

It was my desire that every nurse theorist have a Web presence, so I created a site for Dr. Ernestine Wiedenbach in 1996 that can be found at http://www .clayton.edu/nursing/Nursing-Theory/wiedenbach. I chose to create a site for Wiedenbach because she was a maternal/infant nurse like me and not because I personally used Wiedenbach's theory. It is still my hope that one day every nurse theorist will have a website to increase available information for nurses—even those without ready access to libraries and theory texts. I think many of us, particularly those who live in the United States, can't imagine not having access to information with our extensive library systems and interlibrary loans, and the like. But for many people, particularly those not currently enrolled in an educational program, the availability of information and textbooks can be limited. Access to the Internet is much more widespread than is access to university libraries, underlining the importance of publishing information about theorists on the Internet.

I have also tried to preserve important nursing theory–related information such as Sigma Theta Tau's Memorial to Dr. Virginia Henderson. Sigma Theta Tau hosted on their website Dr. Angela McBride's tribute to Dr. Henderson when the latter passed away, and many websites and libraries linked to it. However, Sigma Theta Tau decided to remove the memorial. To preserve this bit of nursing theory history, I obtained permission from Sigma Theta Tau International to host the tribute to Dr. Henderson in perpetuity on the Eichelberger Nursing Theory website.

Compilation Websites

The history of two nursing theory compilation or repository sites is known. Compilation or repository nursing theory websites are those that list links to existing nursing theory sites rather than directly providing theoretical information. Both compilation sites were established in 1996 and have remained in operation since that time. Other compilation sites have come and gone during the past 20 years, but these two sites have consistently provided information about nursing theory on the Web and responded to seekers of information about nursing theory. The first site is the Nursing Theory Page (NTP; http://www.sandiego.edu/nursing/research/nursing-theory-research.php/). It began on May 21, 1996, and was followed shortly thereafter on November 1, 1996, by the Clayton State University (CSU)/Eichelberger Nursing Theory website (http://www.clayton.edu/nursing/Nursing-Theory).

Both sites were created as a service to the nursing profession to advance the study and use of nursing theory by increasing access to nursing theory knowledge and facilitating connections between nurses interested in using theory in their practice. These services are provided at no cost to the seeker. In the mid-1990s, finding information about nursing theory on the Web was much more difficult than it is today. It is important to remember that in 1996, when the CSU theory site was first started, search engines were much more limited, the now-ubiquitous Google did not even exist, and most webmasters did not understand the ways in which one could lead seekers to a site. A search one day might have yielded entirely different results from one conducted the next day using the same search parameters.

The NTP provides links to multiple nursing theory websites as well as information about theory conferences and other related events (Donnelly, 2001). This website is the collaborative effort of a now-defunct international nursing theory group and is currently supported by the University of San Diego. Judy Norris at the University of Alberta served as the first webmaster for the site until the site was transferred to the servers at the University of San Diego. Ann M. Mayo took over the maintenance of the site. Dr. Mayo still serves as webmaster.

The CSU theory compilation website began as a project of undergraduate students in my Nursing Theory class in the fall of 1996. Understanding the value of facilitating the search for information about nursing theory started by my students, I revamped and expanded the CSU site and have served as the webmaster since the fall of 1996. Clayton State University has provided the server space and support for the site since the beginning.

Managing the CSU Theory Website

I published the Clayton site and have maintained its content and links since its inception. Once the theory website was uploaded, right away I began to receive emails from nursing students from all over the world. All were seeking help in locating resources about the various nurse theorists. It was so exciting to check my inbox and to find inquiries from students, especially those in foreign countries. When I was not able to locate a resource for a student, I always asked the student to share any information he or she came across that would be helpful to others so that I could make it available on the CSU website.

Shortly after publishing the CSU compilation site, I received a rather disconcerting email from one of the members of the international nursing theory group demanding that I immediately take down the website. This individual was very unhappy that another site had been created that led others to theory websites. I was taken aback, to say the least, and for a period of time found myself in a rather heated debate with this member of the NTP community.

After much discussion, we were able to develop a better understanding of the work and purposes of both sites and an appreciation for the contributions that all were making in advancing nursing theory. Webmaster Judy Norris, in particular, was most gracious in acknowledging and helping others in the NTP community realize that no one owned the Internet. And so we did agree that the two sites would cross-list each other's site, share information, and work together.

Several years later, at a Rogerian conference, I had the opportunity to meet the person who wrote the original email telling me to take down my website. We never spoke of the incident.

Lessons Learned

Serving as "web diva" for the CSU site has been a rare opportunity, and it has been a labor of love. The most gratifying aspect of managing the theory website is the privilege of communicating directly with nurse theorists themselves via email and corresponding with students and nurses from all over the world who are interested in theory.

Managing the website has gotten easier over time. The volume of email has lessened as students have become more savvy in searching for information, as sites have become more stable, and as more and more search engines have made searching easier.

I have learned that nursing theorists are, for the most part, very generous people who delight in sharing their knowledge and expertise with others. With the advent of email, seekers have the opportunity to communicate directly with experts in various nursing theories. Some theorists themselves participate in online discussions with seekers. Kathy Kolcaba, Margaret Newman, Savina Schoenhofer, and Imogene King were a few who frequently communicated with students and others about their theories. In 2007, Dr. Imogene King passed away at the age of 84, but until shortly before her death, she routinely answered students' emails.

Lack of permanency of information on the Web remains an area of concern. Because information can be posted one day and removed the next, access to a sizable amount of information is lost over time. I have tried to capture information that I think is particularly useful and that needs to be preserved. I always obtain permission from the original author prior to reposting the information. I then create a new site within my nursing theory site to maintain the information for others. One example is the memorial for Virginia Henderson, originally published on the Sigma Theta Tau website, that I now host on the CSU site. Another example is a paper discussing Johnson's Behavioral System Model. It was removed in 2002 and then reposted on my website (at http://www.clayton.edu/nursing/Nursing-Theory/johnson_behavioral_system).

One of the areas where I see a real need and potential to advance the understanding of nursing theory is that of discussion-based electronic mailing lists or listservs. Listservs are automatic mailing list servers that individuals join with their email addresses. When an email is addressed to a listserv mailing list, it is automatically broadcast to everyone on the list. The result is similar to a newsgroup or forum, except that the messages are transmitted via email and are therefore available only to individuals on the list. Participants routinely post questions in the form of an email blast to the entire listserv membership, and anyone can offer an answer or opinion. Listservs are somewhat time-consuming to maintain, and it is for that reason, I suspect, that many of the theorist groups have abandoned support for them. Parse's group remains the most active electronic mailing list.

Great insights exist in the listserv postings—particularly if the actual theorists and experts who personally worked with the theorists agree to participate. Many of the original theorists are retiring, and many have passed away; the discussions that have occurred on some of the electronic mailing lists contain very valuable explanations and applications but are often lost when the electronic mailing lists are discontinued.

For the first 5 years or so, I did not record the number of hits the CSU site received. Since I began recording, the site has received approximately 1.5 million hits. However, the traffic is decreasing. I believe this is due to the availability of individual proprietary sites; they are ad-generated and diverting potential visitors to advertised sites. My site in not the only site experiencing a decrease in overall numbers of hits per month. The popular Country Joe McDonald Florence Nightingale site has also experienced a slowdown (Tom Weller, personal communication, April 9, 2015). The NTP site reports traffic to their site has remained steady over that past year (Ann Mayo, personal communication, April 22, 2015).

The first 7 years or so, I never received solicitations to advertise on my site; however, years 8 through 13 showed a rise in requests for advertisement and requests for me to add sites for commercial reasons that were not directly related to theory. No advertisements have ever been nor will ever be a part of the CSU nursing theory site. I am very gratified, however, when nurse theorists contact me directly and ask that I add their site to my website and when authors contact me and ask that I list their book or their videos about nursing theory on the site. These requests have decreased during the past 2 years or so.

One of the most fortuitous hits on my site was that of Dr. Kathy Sitzman, my coauthor in writing *Understanding the Work of Nurse Theorists: A Creative Beginning*. Dr. Sitzman and I began a virtual partnership in 2003 that led to the publishing of our text. I received a phone call one day from someone introducing herself as a "lover of nursing theory" and asking whether I would be interested in collaborating with her on a nursing theory textbook. Because of my website, she thought that she would like to work with me. Thus began our long-distance collaboration.

I appreciate having the opportunity to share with you my experiences in serving as webmaster for a nursing theory website. I must say I am very grateful for the class assignment that started it all many years ago. I have long since lost touch with the two students who gave birth to the website, but I want to thank them for giving me the idea that led to one of the most rewarding creative outlets I have had in nursing. It has been a lovely journey.

References

Capra, F. (1975). *The tao of physics*. Retrieved from http://www.plouffe.fr/simon/math/The%20Tao%20of%20Physics.pdf

Donnelly, E. (2001). An assessment of nursing theories as guides to scientific inquiry. In N. L. Chaska (Ed.), *The nursing profession tomorrow and beyond* (p. 332). Thousand Oaks, CA: Sage.

Rogers, M. E. (1970). *An introduction to the theoretical basis of nursing*. Philadelphia, PA: Davis.

Glossary

aesthetics (nursing art) The perception of deep meanings within nursing practice that evoke creativity and result in multilevel understandings and expressions of practice within an artistic context.

assumption Principles that are accepted as being true without proof or concrete verification, usually based on logic, inductive reasoning, or deductive reasoning.

concept An abstraction (thought, model, mental formation) based on the observation of phenomena.

deductive reasoning Formation of specific predictions based on general observations or principles.

domain A territory or field of activity. In nursing practice, generally four domains are recognized: empirics (scientific competence), personal (therapeutic use of self), ethics (moral/ethical comportment), and aesthetics (transformative art/acts).

empirics Replicating, validating, explaining, and structuring. Expressed as knowledge by theories and models and integrated into practice as scientific competence.

ethics A system of moral values that is concerned with "doing the right thing" that is associated with trust, respect, dignity, human/legal rights of the nurse and client and that is based on the consensus of the population involved in the transaction.

grand theory A theory that represents the broad concepts within an entire discipline (e.g., nursing).

hypothesis A statement of a relationship between variables that can be tested.

idea A mental conception or image.

inductive reasoning Formation of general predictions based on specific observations.

knowledge Perception of reality developed through insight, learning, and investigation expressed in a form that can be shared. It is collectively assessed as valuable through shared understanding.

medical model The approach to the diagnosis and treatment of illness as practiced by physicians in the West. The physician focuses on the patient's defect or dysfunction. The medical history, physical examination, and diagnostic tests provide the basis for the identification and treatment of a specific illness or condition.

metaparadigm Refers to an overall worldview (e.g., reductionism, rationalism, relativism). *See also* paradigm.

middle-range theory (practice theory) A theory that focuses on one part of a discipline in an attempt to explain and predict phenomena. Such theories are meant to be directly applicable to everyday nursing practice.

moral/ethical comportment Expression of ethical knowledge and knowing in nursing practice.

nondualism The assertion that everything in the universe is unavoidably interconnected and can never be completely separated into distinct parts. The belief that everything affects everything else to varying degrees.

nursing model A symbolic rendering of ideas or concepts with pictorial elements that illustrates the relationships between and among the ideas or concepts.

nursing process A structured organizational framework for nursing that includes assessment, nursing diagnosis, planning, implementation, and evaluation.

nursing science The systematic exploration, measurement, and explanation of phenomena specific to nursing. Also refers to the body of knowledge that is specific to nursing.

paradigm The lens through which the world is viewed by an individual, group, or discipline. A way of assigning value or worth to observations, knowledge, methods, and phenomena. *See also* metaparadigm.

phenomenon Any event that can be sensed, attended to, or apprehended by a sentient being.

philosophy A system of beliefs about the general nature of things, particularly morality, ethics, and how the world should be viewed. The study of principles underlying human thought, conduct, and understandings about the nature of where we fit in the universe.

postmodern nursing A movement toward knowledge discovery that does not rely exclusively on empirical evidence of phenomena but that also focuses on the discovery of the meaning of phenomena. This is a sort of "learn as you go" approach that is done by immersing oneself in a phenomenon of interest, trying to discern pattern and meaning, while acknowledging the unavoidable interconnectedness of the observer (self) with the phenomenon. *See also* empirics.

research Planned, deliberate study of a specific phenomenon for the purpose of deepening understanding and allowing for prediction and replication of the phenomenon.

scientific medicine Care focused on the illness, not the client. The process of diagnosis depends on structured knowledge that is accepted by the mainstream medical community. Medications, surgeries, and traditional treatments are the focus of practice.

theory An abstract generalization that presents a systematic explanation about the relationships among phenomena. A nursing theory is a theory that is meant to address phenomena specific to nursing practice.

theoretical physics Speculative study and conjecture regarding the interactions, properties, and changes associated with matter and energy.

therapeutic use of self Expression of a personal knowledge and knowing in nursing practice that is integrated with ethics, empiric knowledge, and nursing art.

wholism Being aware of the interaction of many parts, or aspects, that form a whole system.

Index

Note: Page numbers followed by *f* indicate material in figures.

A

activity-related effect, on health-promoting behaviors, 127

adaptation. *See also* Roy Adaptation Model (RAM)

    adaptive responses, 69–73, 81–86

    environmental, 83

    modes of, 82–83

adjustment and healing stress response, 76

advanced beginner skill acquisition stage, Model of Skill Acquisition (Benner), 158

advanced caring–healing modalities/nursing arts, 49

airplane, origami, 106–108, 107*f*

alarm stress response, 76

American Academy of Nursing, 166

American Journal of Nursing, 209

authority, defined, 150

automatic behavior, 113

awareness, transitions property, 170

B

Bandura, Albert, 132

basic conditioning factors, 90

Basic Principles of Nursing Care (Henderson), 36

behavior

    assessment, 84

    automatic, 113

    caring, 160

    coping, 78, 82, 149, 162

    health-promoting, 126–130

    of patients, 112–113

Benner, Patricia

    biographical sketch, 155–156

    skill acquisition in nursing model, 156–162

biological factors, health-promoting, 126
biophysical-medical model, 194
Buddhist mandalas, 66

C

carative factors, 48
care, 98
    defined, 97
    nursing, 91
caring, 98, 205
    carative factors, 48
    caring moments/caring occasions, 49, 51
    caritas processes, 49, 54
    defined, 97, 159
    environment, 52
    global caring field meditation project, 56
    primacy of, 160
    as response to stress, 157
    wholistic caring, 8, 52, 83, 96, 98, 99
caring–healing consciousness, 49
caring moments/caring occasions, 49, 51
Caring Science as Sacred Science (Watson), 55
caritas processes, 49, 54
Cash, K., 206
cathedrals, 66
client/client system, 76–79, 82, 85
clinical caritas processes, 49
clinical nursing, 41–46. *See also* nurse–patient relationship; nursing practice
    clinical caritas processes, 49
    elements of, 42
    key terms, 42–45
    need for help, 43–45
Clinical Nursing: A Helping Art (Wiedenbach), 41
cocreation principle, 197
coexistence, 196
comfort, 117–123. *See also* Theory of Comfort (Kolcaba)
    types of, 118
comfort needs, 119
communication
    information technology, 209–210
    interpersonal systems, 148–149
    in nurse–patient relationship, 138, 145

competent skill acquisition stage, Model of Skill Acquisition (Benner), 158

compilation nursing theory websites, 221–222

compilation sites, 211–212

Complexity Nursing Theory, 214

conceptual systems, 13, 144–145

connectedness, 210

connecting–separating concept, 197

consciousness, 187–189

conservation model (Levine)

    adaptation, 69–73

    assertions, 71

    mandala representation, 71–72

    nursing theories, 69–73

    principles, 71

content sites, 212–213

control, defined, 150

coping, 78, 82, 149, 161–162

cotranscending process, 197–198

CSU nursing theory compilation website, 222–225

cultural and social structure dimensions, 97

cultural care, 97, 98

cultural care accommodation/negotiation, 97

cultural care diversity, defined, 97

cultural care preservation/maintenance, 97

cultural care repatterning/restructuring, 97–98

cultural care universality, 97

cultural diversity, 95–100

culturally congruent care, 96, 98

culture, 97

Culture Care: Diversity and Universality theory (Leininger), 95–100

    culturally congruent care, 96, 98

    mandala representation, 99–100

    wholistic caring, 96, 98, 99

curative vs. carative factors, 48

D

debriefing, 172

decision making, defined, 150

deliberative actions criteria, 113

developmental transitions, 168

diagnosis, nursing, 84, 90, 160

disease/illness, 188
  concept, 183
  defined, 161
  diagnosis, nursing, 84, 90, 160
  prevention, 126
  process, 31
diversity, cultural, 95–100
doctoral nursing programs, 12–13, 15
Dreyfus, Hubert, 156–158
Dreyfus, Stuart, 156–158
Dreyfuses' model, 156–158
Dunn, Halbert, 131
Dynamic Nurse–Patient Relationship, The: Function, Process, and Principles of Professional Nursing Practice (Orlando-Pelletier), 111

E

ease, 118
education, nursing, 12–13, 30, 76
Eichelberger, Lisa Wright
  biographical sketch, 217–219
  nursing theory site, 212, 214
  as Web pioneer, 217–225
enabling–limiting concept, 197
environment
  adaptation, 83
  caring, 52
  comfort, 117–123
  components of, 31
  defined, 77, 183
  environmental paradigm, 146
  personal space, 148
environmental paradigm, 146
evidence-based practice, 133
excessive stimulus, 43
exhaustion stress response, 76
existential philosophy, 194–196
expert skill acquisition stage, Model of Skill Acquisition (Benner), 159

F

feeling of disconnectedness, transitions property, 170
feminist postcolonialism, thought patterns, 168

fluid processes, transitions property, 170
From Novice to Expert: Excellence and Power in Clinical Nursing Practice
    (Benner), 157
full-text journal articles, 209

G

General Adaptation Syndrome, 76
General Systems Theory, 76
global caring field meditation project, 56
global community, 145
goal setting, 84
God
    Nightingale's concept of, 30
    in Roy's model, 85
grand theories, 65–68, 96, 199
Gretebeck, Kimberlee, 132–133
group adaptation, 83

H

health
    in conceptual systems model, 144–145, 147
    in conservation model, 71
    continuum, 77, 85, 199
    defined, 83, 97, 161, 189
    health-promoting behavior, 126–130
    paradigm, 146, 171
    perception of, 65
    as wholistic pattern, 188
Health as Expanding Consciousness theory (Newman), 187–189
    human characteristics, 188
    nursing practice, 188
    as progressive, 179–180
    visualizing, 189
    wholism, 188
health–illness continuum, 77, 85
health paradigm, 146, 171
health-promoting behavior, 126–130
Health-Promotion Model (HPM) (Pender), 125–133, 129*f*
    factors in, 126
    foundational assumptions, 128
    health-promoting behavior, 126–130
    origami representation, 130

help, need for, 42–45

Henderson, Virginia
    biographical sketch, 35–39
    nursing overview, 35–39
    theory in action, 38–39
    Web presence, 221, 224

historicity, 70–72

hospitals, 29, 56, 121–122

Hubble Space Telescope, 180

Human Becoming Theory. *See* Theory of Human Becoming

human beings
    adaptation, 69–73, 76, 83, 85, 131
    basic needs, 37, 43, 82, 90
    becoming, process of, 194–199
    caring exchange participation, 48
    characteristics, 188
    cocreation, 196–198
    comfort needs, 119
    human/beings/persons paradigm, 145–146, 170–171, 182
    human nature, nine assertions about, 182
    human–universe–health process, 199
    person, interpretation of, 160
    self-care, 90–92
    self-concept, 148
    systems model and, 83
    wholistic responses, 119

human/beings/persons paradigm, 145–146, 170–171, 182

human–universe–health process, 199

I

illness. *See* disease/illness

imaging concept, 197

information technology, 209–214
    current uses of, 210–211
    dissemination of, 213–214
    nursing theory websites, 211–213

innovative conceptual system, 181

interdependence adaptation, 83

International Consortium of Parse Scholars, 194

international year of the nurse 2010, 56

Internet, 209–214, 217–225

interpersonal influences, on health-promoting behaviors, 127

Interpersonal Relations in Nursing (Peplau), 137, 139–140

Interpersonal Relations in Nursing theory (Peplau), 137–140

    nurse–patient relationship, 138–140

    nursing, defined, 138

    observations, 138

    origami representation, 140

    practice-based theory development, 14

interpersonal systems, 148–149

intuitive knower, 162

J

Johnson, Dorothy E., 82, 224

K

Kalofissudis, Ioannis A., 214

King, Imogene M., 211

    biographical sketch, 143–151

    conceptual systems, 13, 144–145

    Theory of Goal Attainment, 143–151

    Web presence, 224

Kolcaba, Katharine

    biographical sketch, 117

    reflections, 120–123

    Theory of Comfort, 117–123

    Web presence, 224

L

labyrinths, 66

languaging concept, 196–197

Leininger, Madeleine

    biographical sketch, 95

    Culture Care: Diversity and Universality theory, 95–100

    transcultural nursing, 95–96, 99

Levine, Myra Estrin

    biographical sketch, 69–70

    conservation model, 69–73

listservs, 210–211, 224

lived experiences, thought patterns, 168

Logical Positivism, 15

loving–kindness, 49

Lusk, Sally, 132
Lyon, Pat, 210

M

Magnet status, hospitals, 121–122
man/living/health model, 192. *See also* Theory of Human Becoming
mandalas, 65–68, 68f
    history, 66
    as representational of models/theories, 71–72, 79, 85–86, 92, 99–100
McElmurry, Beverly, 132
Meleis, Afaf Ibrahim
    biographical sketch, 165–167
    Transitions Theory, 167–174
metaparadigms, nursing, 145–147
Meyer, Burton, 167
middle-range theories, 207
    defined, 105
    exploration of, 106, 108
    interpersonal relations, 137–140
    in nursing practice, 105–108
    Theory of Comfort, 117–123
mother–infant bonding for NICU, 8–9
Murray, Edward, 120

N

narrative, personalized inquiry camps, 206
need for help, 42–45, 112–114
Neuman, Betty
    biographical sketch, 75
    systems model, 75–79
Neuman Systems Model, 75–79
    client systems, 76–79
    environment, 77
    interrelated variables, 77–78
    mandala representation, 79
    philosophical base, 76–77
    summary, 77–78
newborn intensive care unit (NICU), 8–9
Newman, Margaret
    biographical sketch, 187
    Health as Expanding Consciousness, 179, 187–189
    Web presence, 224

NICU. *See* newborn intensive care unit

Nightingale, Florence

    biographical sketch, 29–30

    nursing overview, 30–33

    theory development, 12, 13, 30–33, 205, 209

    theory in action, 32–33

    Web presence, 212, 225

    on wholism, 31

nondeliberative behavior, 113

Norris, Judy, 211, 222, 223

Notes on Nursing: What It Is and What It Is Not (Nightingale), 12, 209

novice skill acquisition stage, Model of Skill Acquisition

    (Benner), 157–158

NTP. *See* Nursing Theory Page

nurse theorists, 11–16, 52–56

    use of information technology, 209–214

nurse–patient relationship

    communication, 138, 145

    conservation, 70–72

    culturally congruent care, 96, 98

    as enabling, 160

    evaluation, 84

    help, need for, 42–45, 112–114

    nursing roles, 138–139

    phases, 139

    structure of, 139

    transpersonal caring relationships, 50–51

    wholistic approach, 188

nursing, 97

    defined, 138, 160, 183

    education, 12, 30, 76, 175–176

    goal of, 84, 145

    metaparadigms, 145–147

    paradigm, 146–147, 170

    philosophy, 36

nursing actions, 206

nursing assessment

    behavior, 84

    comfort, 117–123

    mindful, 113

nursing care, 91

    goal of, 71

nursing client, defined, 170–171

Nursing: Concepts of Practice (Orem), 89

Nursing Outlook (Roy), 82

nursing paradigm, 146–147

nursing practice, 9, 25

    clinical nursing, 41–46

    competencies, 162

    concepts used in, 77

    defined, 138, 181

    diagnosis, 84, 90, 160

    evidence-based, 133

    goals, 144–145

    interventions, 90, 121, 132, 137, 183

    key terms, 42–45

    metaparadigms, 145–147

    requirements, essential, 198, 206

    seven domains, 157

    skills, 157–159

    theory, influence on, 7–10

    transcultural, 95–96, 99

    work satisfaction, 122

Nursing Process theory (Orlando-Pelletier), 111–114

    assumptions, 114

    concepts of, 112–113

    need for help, 112–114

    nursing practice, 113–114

    origami representation, 114

    patient behavior, 112–113

nursing research, 8–9, 15. *See also* theories

nursing terminology key terms, 42–45

Nursing: The Philosophy and Science of Caring (Watson), 53

nursing theories, 3–5, 69. *See also* theories

    creators of, 3

    development of, 205–207

    philosophy in, 25

    on Web presence, 220–221

Nursing Theory Page (NTP), 211, 221, 222, 225

O

online communication, 211

operational definitions, 19

Orem, Dorothea
    biographical sketch, 89
    Self-Care model, 89–92
organization
    defined, 150
    purposes of, 4
organizational transitions, 168–169
orientation phase, nurse–patient relationship, 139
origami
    airplane, 106–108, 107f
    art of, 105–108, 108f
    as representational of models/theories, 105–108, 108f, 119–120, 130
    sailboat, 106, 108
Orlando-Pelletier, Ida Jean
    biographical sketch, 111
    nursing process theory, 112–114
outcome patterns transitions, 172

P

Parse-L listserv, 210, 224
Parse, Rosemarie Rizzo
    biographical sketch, 193–194
    theory of human becoming, 194–199
partially compensatory system, 91
patients
    adaptation, 69–73
    basic needs, 37
    behavior, 112–113
    client systems, 76–79, 82, 85
    cultural diversity, 95–100
    defined, 43
    help, need for, 42–45, 112–114
    independence, 38
    physical comfort, 118, 119, 121
    satisfaction ratings, 122–123
Pender, Nola
    biographical sketch, 126–127, 130–133
    Health-Promotion Model, 125–133, 129f
Peplau, Hildegard
    biographical sketch, 137
    Interpersonal Relations in Nursing theory, 14, 137–140
    practice-based theory development, 14

personal factors, health-promoting, 126

personal systems, 147–148

person–environment interaction, 187–188

philosophy

    of caring, 36, 53

    of clinical nursing, 42

    existential, 192–194

    in nursing theory, 25

    philosophical–theoretical framework, 53

    of systems model, 76–77

photography, space, 179–180

physical comfort, 118, 119, 121

physiologic–physical adaptation, 82–83

pointillism, 25–27, 36

postmodern research methods, 15–16

power, defined, 150

powering concept, 197–198

practice-based theory development, 14

presence of milestones, transitions property, 170

prevention, 78, 126, 130

Primacy of Caring, The: Stress and Coping in Health and Illness
    (Benner and Wrubel), 159

primary prevention activities, 78

prior related behavior, health-promoting, 126

process patterns transitions, 174

professional activities, 25

professional nursing actions, 113

proficient skill acquisition stage, Model of Skill Acquisition
    (Benner), 158–159

psychological factors, health-promoting, 126

psychospiritual comfort, 118, 119

Q

qualitative data, 72

quantitative data, 72

R

RAM. *See* Roy Adaptation Model

redundancy, 70–72

reflective practice, 14

relief, 118

repository nursing theory websites, 221–222

research, 8–9, 12, 15
resistance and adaptation stress response, 76
revealing–concealing concept, 197
Robbins, Lorraine, 132–133
Rogers, Martha
    biographical sketch, 181
    Unitary Human Beings theory, 13, 179, 181–184, 187, 194
role function adaptation, 83
role theory, thought patterns, 168
roles, 83, 138–139, 149
Roy Adaptation Model (RAM), 81–86
    client systems, 82, 85
    major concepts, 83–84
    mandala representation, 85–86
    nursing process, 84
    scientific/philosophical assumptions, 84–86
Roy, Callista
    Adaptation Model, 81–86
    biographical sketch, 81–82

S

sailboat, origami, 106, 108
Schoenhofer, Savina, 224
Science of Unitary Human Being (Rogers), 219
scientific, structured inquiry camps, 206
Sechrist, Karen, 132
secondary prevention activities, 78
self-care, 90–92
self-care agency, 90
self-care deficit, 91
Self-Care model (Orem), 89–92
    mandala representation, 92
    nursing process steps, 91–92
    nursing systems, 91
    primary needs, 90
    self-care concepts, 90–92
    self-care deficit, 91
    supportive-educative system, 91
self-concept group identity adaptation, 83
Seurat, Georges, 25–28
Sigma Theta Tau's Memorial, 221
situation concept, 161

situational influences, on health-promoting behaviors, 127

situational transitions, 168

Sitzman, Kathy, 225

skill acquisition in nursing model (Benner), 155–162

    concepts, 159

    nursing, defined, 160

    stages, 157–159

    theoretical influences, 156

social systems, 149–150

sociocultural comfort, 118–120

sociocultural factors, health-promoting, 126

space photography, 179–180

specificity, 70–72

status, defined, 150

stimuli assessment, 84

stress

    coping, 149, 161–162

    defined, 149, 161

    responses, 76, 157

Stromborg, Marilyn, 132

structuring meaning, 196, 197

supportive–educative system, 91

systems

    client, 76–79, 82, 85

    conceptual, 13, 144–145

    defined, 82

    interpersonal, 148–149

    nursing, 91

    personal, 147–148

    social, 149–150

T

termination phase, nurse–patient relationship, 139

tertiary prevention activities, 78

theories

    in action, 32–33

    categories, 4–5, 179–180

    components of, 20

    development/evolution, 7–10, 205–207

    evaluation, 19–21

    grand theories, 65–68, 96, 199

    information technology and, 209–214

middle-range theories, 105–108, 117–123

nursing, 3–5

operational definitions, 19

philosophy in, 25–27

reflective practice, 14

research influences, 8, 15

testing of, 15–16

theoretical definitions, 19

valuable aspects of, 207

Web presence, 211–213, 217–225

theorists, 11–16

Theory of Comfort (Kolcaba), 117–123

assumptions, 119

comfort, defined, 118

documentation, 121

origami representation, 119–120

reflections, 120–123

Theory of Goal Attainment (King), 143–151

assumptions, 145–147

conceptual framework, 150–151

conceptual systems, 144–145

learning, defined, 148

system interaction, 148–149

time perception, 148

Theory of Human Becoming (Parse), 194–199

basic beliefs/assumptions, 195–196

existential philosophy, 194–196

as grand theory, 199

human–universe–health process, 199

man/living/health model, 194

nursing requirements, 198

Parse-L mailing list, 210, 224

principles, 196–198

Theory of Human/Transpersonal Caring (Watson), 47–52

caring-healing consciousness, 49

caring moments/caring occasions, 49, 51

caritas processes, 49, 54

major elements, 49–51

transpersonal caring relationships, 50–51

therapeutic self-care demand, 90

time span, transitions property, 170

Toward a Theory for Nursing: General Concepts of Human Behavior (King, 1971), 143 transactions, defined, 149

transcendence, 118

transcultural nursing, 95–96, 99

transforming process, 198

Transitions Theory (Meleis), 165–174

    assumptions, 169

    basic belief, 168

    clinical applications, 172–173

    definition, 168–169

    interventions, 172

    nursing education, 173–174

    nursing practice, 170

    overview, 167–168

    properties/concepts, 169–171

    responses to transitions, 172

transpersonal caring relationships, 50–51

Travis, John, 131

Turner, Ralph H., 167

U

Unitary Human Beings theory (Rogers), 181–184

    assertions, 182, 187–188, 194

    development, 13

    as ground breaking, 219

    key terms, 182–183

    nursing actions, 183

    as progressive, 179–180

    summary, 183–184

universality, 97

V

valuing concept, 197

Van Sell, Sharon L., 214

W

Walker, Susan, 132

Watson Caring Science Institute, 56

Watson, Jean

    biographical sketch, 52–56

    Theory of Human/Transpersonal Caring, 47–52

Websites, 211–213, 221–225

Weller, Tom, 212–213

wellness
  concepts, 76, 183
  perception of, 19, 65, 131
wholism
  concept of, 31, 183–184, 188
  cultural diversity, 95–100
  in nursing practice, 52
  in system theory, 76
wholistic care, concept of, 7–8
wholly compensatory system, 91
Wiedenbach, Ernestine, 220–221
  biographical sketch, 41–45
  clinical nursing, 41–46
working phase, nurse–patient relationship, 139
World Wide Web (WWW)
  information impermanency, 224
  nursing theories, presence of, 211–213, 217–225
worldview, defined, 97
Wrubel, Judith, 157, 159–162
WWW. *See* World Wide Web